Bioethics in Social Context

Bioethics
in Social Context

Edited by

BARRY HOFFMASTER

TEMPLE UNIVERSITY PRESS
Philadelphia

Temple University Press, Philadelphia 19122
Copyright © 2001 by Temple University
All rights reserved
Published 2001
Printed in the United States of America

⊗ The paper used in this publication meets the requirements of the American National
Standard for Information Sciences—Permanence of Paper for Printed Library Materials,
ANSI Z39.48-1984

Library of Congress Cataloging-in-Publication Data

Bioethics in social context / edited by Barry Hoffmaster.
     p. cm.
   Includes biographical references and index.
    ISBN 1-56639-844-4 (cloth : alk. paper)—ISBN 1-56639-845-2 (pbk. : alk. paper)
     1. Medical ethics—Social aspects. 2. Ethnography—Moral and ethical aspects.
   3. Bioethics. 4. Bioethics. I. Hoffmaster, C. Barry.
   R724.B4826 2001
   174'.2—dc21   00-055213

Contents

Acknowledgments

The chapters in this volume are the culmination of three meetings of the Humanizing Bioethics research group that were held in London, Ontario. We are very grateful to the Social Sciences and Humanities Research Council of Canada for supporting this project and making this book possible (grant 806-93-0051). I am also grateful to the staff of the Westminster Institute for Ethics and Human Values (now defunct) for their assistance throughout this project, and in particular to Jean Dalgleish and Marilyn Newman for the customarily professional manner in which they organized the meetings of the research group and made sure they ran smoothly. I thank Wendy Palmer for preparing the manuscript proficiently and efficiently. I thank Susan Bentley for her speedy and scrupulous indexing and for her keen proofreading. And I thank Michael Ames for his abiding interest in and enthusiasm about this collection and for his editorial acumen.

Bioethics in Social Context

BARRY HOFFMASTER

Introduction

BIOETHICS HAS been preoccupied with making judgments about troublesome moral problems and justifying those judgments, with doing what has been aptly called "quandary ethics."[1] Following the lead of philosophical ethics, justification is regarded as a matter of providing "good reasons" for judgments, and that, in turn, is taken to require an appeal to moral rules or principles or to moral theories. Bioethics, in this view, is situated in rationality and generality. It prescinds the messy details and attachments that give our lives meaning and vigor, the nagging contradictions that make us squirm and struggle, and the social, political, and economic arrangements that simultaneously create and constrain us. Because they are yoked to the abstractions of reason and theory, judgments about matters of bioethics frequently outstrip the contexts that generate and shape those matters and ignore the agonizing experiences of the people who grapple with them.

Given the emphasis on theoretical justification in bioethics, it is no surprise that social scientists have remained at its margins. Justifying decisions or judgments is the concern of *normative* ethics, and normative ethics is about what *ought* to be the case—what decision ought to be made, what action ought to be taken, what policy ought to be adopted. *Descriptive* ethics, in contrast, is "the factual investigation of moral behavior and beliefs" (Beauchamp and Childress 1994:4–5). Social scientists—anthropologists, sociologists, and historians—engage in descriptive ethics when they investigate and interpret the actual moral beliefs, codes, or practices of a society or culture, but such nonnormative work is regarded as "secondary to the enterprise of normative ethics" (Beauchamp and Childress 1979:9) and thus secondary to the enterprise of bioethics.[2]

This volume has two related goals: to show that bioethics is as much about *understanding* as it is about *justification,* and to give social scientists a prominent position in a reoriented bioethics. Indeed, it would seem that understanding has to accompany, if not precede, any genuine form of justification, so that, contrary to the prevailing view, what social scientists can tell us is neither independent of nor ancillary to the enterprise of bioethics.

In fact, the interpretations of moral life and moral phenomena provided by social scientists reveal that a rigorous separation of the descriptive and the normative is practically untenable. A dichotomy between the descriptive and the normative (or between fact and value, "is" and "ought") seems to be simply an artifact of the theoretical project of justification, not an intrinsic feature of moral experience.

How, though, is moral understanding to be acquired? One important ingredient of that understanding is an appreciation of the contexts within which moral matters arise and are addressed. Putting bioethics in personal, social, and cultural contexts opens the way for modes of moral deliberation that are not general, rational, and impartial but that embrace the distinctive histories, relationships, and milieus of people and engage their emotions as much as their reason. Such a bioethics also recognizes the multiple backgrounds—institutional, economic, historical, and political—that structure moral problems and give meaning to moral concepts. This is a bioethics situated in lived human experience. The qualitative research approaches of the social sciences, ethnography in particular, can be used to explore the moral dimensions of that experience and thus to enhance our understanding of the nature of morality and its place in our lives. The ultimate goal of this endeavor is a bioethics that is more attuned to the particular and more sensitive to the personal—a bioethics that is more humane and more helpful.

But, the skeptic will insist, even if this call is appealing in the abstract, what does it mean in practice? How would a bioethics more influenced by social scientists and more directed to understanding be different from and better than the existing version? To suggest how that question should be answered requires a survey of what social science forays into bioethics have already produced.

FOUR SOCIAL SCIENCE EXAMPLES

The justificatory apparatus of traditional bioethics: (i) assumes that real-life moral problems come sorted, labeled, and ready for the manipulation of rules, principles, or theories; (ii) disregards the extent to which moral concepts and norms derive their meaning and their force from the social and cultural surroundings in which they are embedded; (iii) neglects the ways in which moral problems are generated and framed by the practices, structures, and institutions within which they arise;

and (iv) ignores the means by which social and cultural ideologies, and the power relationships they entrench, can both perpetuate moral inertia and effect moral change. Kaufman's (1997) study of how medical responsibility is constructed in geriatric medicine, Gordon and Paci's (1997) investigation of the nondisclosure of cancer diagnoses and prognoses in Italy, Anspach's (1987, 1993) examination of neonatal intensive care, and Lock's research on menopause (1993) and reproductive technologies (1998) in Japan address, respectively, these four failings.

Kaufman's interviews of physicians who practice geriatric medicine tellingly reveal that there is no clear demarcation between the moral and the clinical. One cannot focus exclusively on the clinical aspects of a problem at one moment, then shift exclusively to the moral aspects at another moment because, as Kaufman concludes, problems are "irreducibly 'clinically-moral'" (1997:20). That irreducibility complicates the very identification of moral problems and raises questions about what the upshot of labeling a problem "moral" ultimately is.

A troubling clinical-moral issue for every health care professional is determining the boundaries of responsibility. An inner-city internist whom Kaufman interviewed related a story about a seventy-nine-year-old woman who cares for her twelve-year-old grandson and nine-year-old granddaughter because her son is a homeless heroin addict. The grandchildren's mother, who was also a heroin addict, is dead. Because the grandmother is becoming progressively more demented, it is not clear how much longer she can care for her grandchildren. Her son is a patient of the internist, but the grandmother is not. The grandmother participates in the Grandparents Who Care program at the internist's public health center, though, and the internist facilitated a support group to which the grandmother belonged. The internist also has done respite care for the family and has taken the children on outings. Even though the grandmother is not an official patient, she is someone the internist "cares about, feels an obligation toward, and 'treats' in the context of a grandparent support group which she started because so many patients (and family members) need psychological and material, as well as medical, support" (1997:11). The internist agonizes about the boundaries of her medical and personal responsibility and even goes so far as to consider adopting the two children. Kaufman summarizes what is at stake here:

> The dominant theme of the tale is the problem of how to ensure the well-being of the entire family. Adoption as a potential solution to the

dilemma-tale projects a moral self who ponders and problematizes the role of physician: if she cannot give what she considers to be adequate or optimal care *as a doctor*, perhaps she could—and should—become *family* in order to create a substitute for the "missing" middle generation. Stepping into that space herself as both concerned parent and child would, in her view, get to the crux of the problem. (1997:11–12; emphasis in original)

This is not a typical bioethics problem. To some, it might not even be a recognizable bioethics problem, yet it concerns the fundamental matter of medical-moral responsibility and the clinical-moral issues of who is a patient and what should be treated. The internist's dilemma shows how clinically entangled and fluid is the notion of the moral. Given the mutuality and the irreducibility of the clinical and the moral, the content of bioethics cannot be segregated in a set of normative principles and rules that are brought to bear on the factual goings-on of the clinic.

Gordon and Paci's study of concealment and silence around cancer in Italy reveals how deeply and widely the values and beliefs pertinent to bioethics are embedded in social and cultural ways of being. At the particular, individual level Gordon and Paci trace Dr. J.'s practice of not informing patients of diagnoses and prognoses to the practices of not telling and not knowing that he learned before entering medicine and that he employed in a variety of situations. Reflecting on his upbringing, Dr. J. relates a general lesson he was taught: "If someone had a problem that bothers him, we were brought up to keep it inside, to not say anything about it, because you are sorry to involve others in this suffering, especially if there is nothing they can do about it" (1997:1445). And a description of the common practice of "parents waiting to leave until a child is distracted or using little lies to cover up or ease a separation or pain," strikes a chord with Dr. J.: "Yes, yes, they teach you early on to lie, from childhood. That sounds right! I learned that's how it is. You mustn't say things as they are. You are better for it, I am better for it!" (1997:1445) Although Dr. J.'s biography is idiosyncratic, Gordon and Paci report that "it echoes themes heard repeatedly in other accounts . . . and draws upon common cultural and social resources shared to varying extents by people of the same age, gender, class, city, region, country, and religion that together constitute the cultural field of this local world" (1997:1445). Moreover, what goes on in health care manifests those "common cultural and social resources":

[C]oncealment, silence or ambiguity are not just practices of protection from death and illness in the health sector but also ways of keeping problems and emotions "private" and out of the social arena, of avoiding conflict, disobedience and punishment, of asserting autonomy for the dominated . . . of coping by avoiding facing problems or painful topics, of expressing love, protecting another, and being responsible by sparing others' suffering. (1997:1445–1446)

Those shared practices and understandings are, Gordon and Paci argue, "embedded in and contribute to the construction and reconstruction of larger meta-narratives" about matters such as personhood, individuality and sociality, hierarchy, time, and the good life (1997:1447). Their exploration of the background to the nondisclosure of cancer diagnoses and prognoses leads Gordon and Paci to conclude:

[O]ne senses a strong social field or force opertive [sic] in this context, one that effectively creates reality, that defines morality, that can make people comply, that can pass on emotions, that can pull one out of sorrow through distraction. . . . This strong social field works on open, socially porous, "suggestable," [sic] "fragile" people and ways of being-in-the-world. (1997:1448)

That shared social background is what injects morality with practical meaning and force, what gives morality the significance it has in our lives.

Moral problems are, as well, a function of institutional and structural factors, as Anspach's study of neonatal intensive care demonstrates. Anspach found that a consensus around moral principles does not remove controversy about the treatment of seriously ill newborns because doctors and nurses frequently disagree about the prognoses for these infants. Those discrepant prognostic judgments result from the different work experiences that doctors and nurses have. Doctors, who spend relatively little time with the infants in a neonatal intensive care unit (NICU), base their conclusions on physical findings, the results of diagnostic tests, and the literature of medical research. Nurses, who spend concentrated and extended periods of time with these infants, rely on their personal and social interactions with the infants. There is, as a result, a clash between what Anspach calls the different "modes of knowing" of the two groups (1987:227).

Those two modes of knowing, Anspach discovered, emanate from how work is divided and organized within an NICU. Because attending physicians visit the unit for brief periods of time, because house staff rotate through the unit on short cycles, and because physicians in tertiary care institutions often have research interests, doctors are both organizationally and personally detached from these infants and their parents. The information they rely on to formulate a problem and resolve it is the technical and, in the case of research findings, general information they possess and value. Because nurses, in contrast, are intimately and continuously involved with the care of these infants, they are organizationally and personally attached to them. Their perceptions of problems and their responses to them arise from their interactions with the infants.

But, as Anspach also observes, the "technological cues" of the doctors and the "interactive cues" of the nurses are not valued equally: "[T]he interactive cues noted by the nurses are *devalued data*" (1987:229; emphasis in original). Why is that? One obvious answer ties the devaluation of the nurses' data to prevailing gender roles in society. Another answer, offered by Anspach, appeals to the history of diagnostic technology and locates newborn intensive care in a "postclinical" medical culture, that is, a culture in which the science of medicine has displaced the art of medicine. In such a scientistic culture, the soft "subjective" information of the nurses is no match for the hard, "objective" data of the doctors. From beginning to end, the moral disagreement between the doctors and the nurses is framed and settled by factors well beyond the confines of traditional bioethics.

Lock's research on menopause and reproductive technologies in Japan reveals how deeply and how intractably moral beliefs and values can be embedded in cultural backgrounds suffused with unexamined assumptions and unequal power relationships. In Japan, for instance, a dominant moral ideology dictates that women should stay at home and raise their children because this practice is "natural" and because women are biologically programmed to nurture others. Women who use babysitters other than their own mothers are frowned upon. As well, the Japanese government and medical profession do not promote artificial insemination with donor sperm or any form of surrogate motherhood because a dominant moral ideology holds that biological and social parenting should coincide and that these reproductive technologies threaten notions of the family and correct parenting that must remain inviolate. Many Japanese women, not just committed feminists, are familiar with theories of autonomy and Western feminist ideas.

They also know that their society puts the family first, and they usually have many doubts about "the West" and its devotion to individualism and autonomy. They recognize that the dominant ideology in Japan values communalism and family, and they recognize that this ideology has drawbacks; but they do not, by any means, fully support American or French feminism or wish it on Japanese women. They are acutely aware of these tensions, just as they are aware that their government has a moral agenda for Japanese women.

Appraising the moral plight and reactions of Japanese women requires an understanding of the extent to which dominant, culturally infused ideologies are congruent with everyday practices and why congruence, or the lack thereof, exists. Are these ideologies internalized to such an extent that people do not even recognize them as troubling or do not resist them? Or do they ignore them or actively work against them? Qualitative research methods such as ethnography can suggest some answers. Ethnography can tease apart relationships among cultural traditions, power, and emerging and existing ideologies, and it can illuminate what is "normal," "natural," and "right" among particular groups in discrete circumstances and where ruptures and tensions exist among values. When morality is situated in experience, it cannot be severed from the seamless heterogeneity of that experience, and understanding morality *as it is lived* shows how intimately it is intertwined with culturally grounded knowledge, power, institutions, and practices.

The chapters in this volume explore the themes that these four examples illustrate. They show how bioethics problems are the product of institutional, social, historical, and cultural contexts and how power gets wielded within those contexts. They reveal how strikingly absent contextual considerations can be from the work of bioethics and how that absence gets in the way of good bioethics. They render those who have to make and live with moral decisions more visible. The chapters strive to broaden bioethics beyond the theoretical confines within which it largely operates. They also strive to connect bioethics more closely to people's lives and the situations in which moral problems arise. But this volume is only a first step on an exploratory journey. The chapters suggest what the destination could be and point toward that destination. The motivation for embarking on this journey is the prospect of a bioethics that is more realistic and more helpful.

PRACTICAL IMPLICATIONS

Putting bioethics in context should have important practical implications. For one thing, this enterprise could expose gaps between theory and practice and explain why the achievements of bioethics have sometimes been modest and even disappointing. For example, although bioethics emphasizes respecting the autonomy of patients and their families and obtaining informed consent, those goals are imperfectly realized at best. Anspach reports that "although professionals in both intensive-care nurseries I studied acknowledged the importance of involving the parents in the decision-making process, an assent model, rather than an informed consent paradigm, was most frequently used" (1993:92). Moreover, the assent that was given could, of course, be manufactured by "slanting" the clinical information presented to parents (1993:96). And Anspach found that departures from the ideal of informed parental consent were not haphazard: "[I]n both nurseries . . . the decision-making process was organized so as to limit parents' options—even to the extent of eliminating them from some decisions altogether. The actual, if sometimes unstated, aim of the conference with parents was to elicit their agreement to decisions staff had already made" (1993:95–96).

Sociologists who have studied the medical care of adults reach similar conclusions. Robert Zussman found that informed consent played "only a small role" in the two intensive care units in which he did his fieldwork (1992:83). Daniel Chambliss's observation is even more sobering: "In major medical centers, 'informed consent' represents at best a polite fiction" (1993:651). Why and how does such a discrepancy between theory and practice exist?

Zussman's study of intensive care (1992) provides one answer. Those in positions of power in a hospital can subvert the theoretical goals of bioethics through conceptual gerrymandering. Vesting decision-making authority in patients has put physicians in the uncomfortable position of having to do things they believe are professionally or morally wrong, but when physicians get pushed too far, they resist. Zussman describes how:

> In stressing physicians' resistance to the wishes of patients and families, I do not question the sincerity with which they accept patients' legitimate priority in matters bearing on values. Physicians do not typically defend their discretion by claiming explicit jurisdiction over such matters. Indeed,

physicians rarely question the values of their patients. . . . Rather, when physicians do resist the wishes of patients and their families, they justify that resistance by moving decisions from the realm of values to the realm of technique. Thus, physicians argue, frequently and insistently, that some decisions are not value laden at all but simply technical. As such, many physicians argue, they are beyond the proper range not only of patients and families but of both the law and ethics more generally. (1992:141–142)

Nowhere is that strategy clearer than with the controversial but clinically well-entrenched notion of futility. Physicians can parry the demand to "do everything" for a critically ill patient on the basis of their "technical" judgment that further treatment would be "futile." That is an inviting strategy because "a technical judgment raises no issues of values and requires no consultation with family or friends. Ethics is transformed into medicine" (Zussman 1992:151).

Anspach's and Zussman's studies of intensive care show how moral prescriptions about what ought to be done can be blocked by the decision-making procedures and the power relationships that exist in a hospital. Instituting moral and social change consequently requires more than education and rational argument and persuasion (see Jennings 1990). Putting bioethics in context helps to expose the institutional, social, and cultural forces that create gaps between theory and practice and points bioethics in directions that are more likely to produce moral reform.

At the same time, though, putting bioethics in context could have sobering consequences for those who engage in bioethics. Perhaps surprisingly given his own life and writings, Milan Kundera characterizes the novel as "a *realm where moral judgment is suspended.* Suspending moral judgment is not the immorality of the novel; it is its *morality.* The morality that stands against the ineradicable human habit of judging instantly, ceaselessly, and everyone; of judging before, and in the absence of, understanding. From the viewpoint of the novel's wisdom, that fervid readiness to judge is the most detestable stupidity, the most pernicious evil" (1995:7; emphasis in original).

It would be foolish to suggest that patients, their families, and health care professionals abstain from making moral judgments. It would be equally foolish and irresponsible to suggest that practitioners of bioethics judge "instantly, ceaselessly, and everyone." But it is not foolish to suggest that the judgments of right and wrong so common in and expected of bioethics should be made more cautiously and more circumspectly, that suspending moral judgment might often be the morality, not the immorality, of bioethics. For the judgments of bioethics need to rest on more than philosophically respectable "good reasons"—they need to proceed from and manifest an understanding of morality as lived human experience. That bioethics can come to embrace that kind of understanding is the hope of this volume.

NOTES

Acknowledgments: I thank Sharon Kaufman and Margaret Lock for their generosity with their time, their acute critical comments, their direction, their contributions, and their encouragement. This chapter is immeasurably better as a result of their help.

1. This approach is not only because of the nature of the field but also because of the analytic philosophical tradition that has so strongly influenced contemporary bioethics. See, for example, "Quandary Ethics" in Pincoffs 1986:13–36.

2. This quotation from the first edition of *Principles of Biomedical Ethics* is deleted in the three subsequent editions. In those succeeding editions, though, the authors continue to insist that they are concerned primarily with normative ethics. The distinction between normative ethics and descriptive ethics is an article of faith for those who come to bioethics from a philosophical background. In his examination of the just distribution of health care services, Daniels, for example, explains: "I will concern myself with what I think ought to be the case and not just with what a moral anthropologist surveying our practice might discover is the case" (1985:116).

REFERENCES

Anspach, Renee R. 1987. Prognostic Conflict in Life-and-Death Decisions: The Organization as an Ecology of Knowledge. *Journal of Health and Social Behavior* 28:215–231.

———. 1993. *Deciding Who Lives.* Berkeley: University of California Press.

Beauchamp, Tom L., and James F. Childress. 1979. *Principles of Biomedical Ethics.* New York: Oxford University Press.

———. 1994. *Principles of Biomedical Ethics,* 4th ed. New York: Oxford University Press.

Chambliss, Daniel F. 1993. Is Bioethics Irrelevant? *Contemporary Sociology* 22:649–652.

Daniels, Norman. 1985. *Just Health Care.* Cambridge: Cambridge University Press.

Gordon, Deborah R., and Eugenio Paci. 1997. Disclosure Practices and Cultural Narratives: Understanding Concealment and Silence around Cancer in Tuscany, Italy. *Social Science and Medicine* 44:1433–1452.

Jennings, Bruce. 1990. Ethics and Ethnography in Neonatal Intensive Care. In *Social Science Perspectives on Medical Ethics,* ed. George Weisz, 261–272. Boston, MA: Kluwer Academic.

Kaufman, Sharon R. 1997. Construction and Practice of Medical Responsibility: Dilemmas and Narratives from Geriatrics. *Culture, Medicine and Psychiatry* 21:1–26.

Kundera, Milan. 1995. *Testaments Betrayed,* trans. Linda Asher. New York: HarperCollins.

Lock, Margaret. 1993. *Encounters with Aging: Mythologies of Menopause in Japan and North America.* Berkeley: University of California Press.

————. 1998. Perfecting Society: Reproductive Technologies, Genetic Testing, and the Planned Family in Japan. In *Pragmatic Women and Body Politics,* eds. Margaret Lock and Patricia A. Kaufert, 206–239. Cambridge: Cambridge University Press.

Pincoffs, Edmund L. 1986. *Quandaries and Virtues.* Lawrence: University Press of Kansas.

Zussman, Robert. 1992. *Intensive Care.* Chicago: University of Chicago Press.

Sharon R. Kaufman

1   Clinical Narratives and Ethical Dilemmas in Geriatrics

By now the critique of traditional bioethics, based on tenets of Western philosophical rationalist thought (Marshall 1992), is well known in the medical social sciences. Clinicians and others have commented on the remoteness or ineffectiveness of moral theory for actual problem solving (Anspach 1993; Hoffmaster 1992, 1994; Smith and Churchill 1986). Social scientists have noted the lack of attention to culture, ethnicity, and economics in North American bioethics and the primacy it grants individualism and self-determination as these notions have emerged in the Western (predominantly Anglo-American) industrialized world (Fox 1991; Kleinman 1995; Marshall 1992).

Ethnographers studying physician training (Bosk 1979; Muller 1992; Muller and Koenig 1988), the doctor-patient relationship (Good et al. 1990; Gordon 1990; Taylor 1988), decision making in a variety of medical contexts (Anspach 1993; Bosk 1992; Clark, Potter, and McKinlay 1991), and the impact of new technologies on patient care and values in medicine (Fox and Swazey 1992: Kaufman 1993; Koenig 1988) are broadening the conceptual boundaries of ethical inquiry by delineating a range of dilemmas in clinical practice from a grounded, empirical point of view. Their detailed studies of local situations, attention to structural, cultural, and political sources of dilemmas, and analyses of moral problems from patient and practitioner viewpoints show the limitations of existing moral theory for understanding the scope and complexity of dilemmas that physicians, patients, and families actually face. This chapter adds to the growing ethnographic literature on the nature of dilemmas in medical practice through an exploration of narratives as modes of clinical–moral reasoning[1] in the field of geriatrics.

Through analyzing narrative accounts of dilemmas in geriatric medicine, this chapter illustrates how one dimension of bioethics is the "lived experience"[2] of physicians whose stories of primary care are morally problematic for them. The intent of this chapter is to contribute to the conversation among social scientists and medical ethicists about what constitutes ethical concern and activity in actual medical practice and what methods best access that concern. It uses two strategies. First, it opens the *content* of bioethics to a range of underdiscussed topics (such as risk, sufficient action, and the ambiguity of "comfort care") that physicians in geriatrics cite as deeply troubling. Second, it expands the *nature* of bioethics beyond rational ethical deliberation per se to show that clinical-moral deliberation and actual problem solving are dynamic activities situated both in local worlds where explicit institutional structures, demands, and expectations shape practices, and in broader contexts of cultural discourse and debate, ideology, and value that more tacitly frame the knowledge, construction, and understanding of medical problems and their potential solutions.

In addition, this chapter pays attention to two conceptual concerns of social scientists interested in further articulating the ethical dimensions of medical practice. First, awareness of the multiple contexts of health care delivery—not only the physical setting of the acute care hospital—is essential for understanding the range of physicians' ethical concerns. Bioethics as both a profession and a social representation of public distress over expanding medical authority emerged in the United States from troubled decision making about the use of technology in the hospital. Much bioethics debate continues to focus on conflicts between life prolongation and attendant suffering, on the one hand, and "comfort," pain reduction, and "dignity," on the other. Yet doctor-patient interactions, wherever they occur physically, are situated also in structural, political, and socioeconomic environments that influence the construction of clinical-moral problems. Sources of dilemmas are in many cases beyond the literal walls of hospital, clinic, home, and office and are located, more importantly, in the organization and financing of health care delivery, the press to make use of intensive care units and nursing homes, the perceived "need" to utilize the newest technologies, the priority on action, and other features of the cultural field in which physicians practice (Fox 1991; Rhodes 1993). Socioeconomic and cultural features have been neglected or devalued in the construction of bioethics as a profession and applied discipline.

Second, the notion of an autonomous and completely unencumbered individual (in this case the doctor) as the locus of responsibility for therapeutic choice (Kleinman 1995; Koenig 1993) is misguided. Various social scientists have shown how the locus of responsibility for moral choice making is embedded in structural features of medical practice, institutional priorities, social characteristics of the physician and patient, and in shifting and interlinked power relations among individual players (Anspach 1993; Bosk 1992; Clark, Potter, and McKinlay 1991; Hoffmaster 1992; Lindenbaum and Lock 1993). Actual decision making often is not a deliberate, rational, or autonomous act on the part of an individual clinician, as bioethical theory would have it. In fact, decisions are not always "made" in an active, premeditated sense. Rather, they sometimes "happen" as events unfold. "Decisions" actually encompass a variety of practices, some articulated as conscious choice making, others taken for granted as routine steps in an undifferentiated process of clinical activity. Thus decisions may emerge during negotiations with patients, family members, other health professionals, and agency or institutional representatives. They may occur without overt discussion. They may evolve slowly and, at times, invisibly.

Even when decision making is an explicit act, it can be a murky enterprise. Doctors who were subjects in an anthropological study of ethical dilemmas in geriatrics[3] reported that they often do not know what the best clinical-moral choice is among a range of care options, yet they usually feel compelled to be active and do something. Their choices, gauged from the vantage point of the supreme value placed on action in the service of diagnosis, management, and cure, are not always comfortable for them. The discomfort and tension that exist between individual professional sensibilities and quandaries about care, respect, and the purposes of medical intervention, on the one hand, and the structural pressure to institutionalize and use the technological armamentarium available, on the other, are not recognized in theoretical, analytical, principle-based bioethics.

Method: The Use of Narrative

Narrative, used here in a limited sense to refer to accounts or stories that relate subjective experiences, the unfolding of events or conversation, and causal explanations, has been increasingly employed in the last few years by scholars and clinicians who seek to extend the boundaries of bioethical understanding to include socioeconomic conditions, everyday practices, and the impacts of cultural trends on medical knowledge, practice, and uncertainty. Toward this end narrative, as both method and text, has been invoked in the following ways: to describe patient-centered perspectives of illness and suffering, including patients' moral worlds (Frank 1995; Good 1994; Kleinman 1988; Kleinman and Kleinman 1991); to understand the process of clinical judgment, the evaluation of treatment choices, and the incommensurability of physician and patient reasoning (Hunter 1991); to illustrate how actors in medical scenarios frame intentionality (Mattingly 1994) and time (Good et al. 1994); to discern what is "good" for patients (Mattingly 1991, 1993; Smith and Churchill 1986); to investigate power relations between patients and providers (Mishler 1984; Waitzkin 1991); and, generally, to give weight to the gender, life stories, and cultural identities of moral agents, whose unique, contextualized perspectives and positions have been ignored or muted in traditional bioethics (Frank 1995; Pellegrino 1994). Advocates of narrative argue that, as a method, it captures and constitutes both lived morality and experience and the dynamics of social practices and conditions, thus revealing an open, richer field of ethical reasoning and ethical behavior than abstract perspectives allow (Muller 1994).

Here I use narratives drawn from interviews I conducted with physicians who treat older patients: (1) to explore tensions and ambiguities in geriatric medical practice—as well as the cultural sources of those tensions—that may not be revealed through other approaches; (2) to give voice to the lived, practical concerns of the most powerful players in the health care arena; and (3) to look for relationships between "culture" and "ethics" that are embedded in this particular form of cultural expression.

The Study and Sample

The interviews are part of a larger investigation of physician conceptualizations that underlie clinical-ethical decision making in geriatrics. Thus the stories physicians told were both deliberately solicited and consciously and reflectively offered.[4] The important inclusion criterion for the study was clinicians' experience with an elderly population. Twenty-nine of fifty-one physicians treated mainly persons over sixty-five (60 percent to 100 percent of their patients). The other twenty-two physicians noted that 20 percent to 50 percent of their patients were elderly. This was a convenience sample generated by "snowball" techniques. I began by interviewing several internists and family practitioners known to me. At the end of those interviews, I asked for the names of other physicians who treat elderly patients. Those individuals were asked also to recommend colleagues to be interviewed. I made every attempt to solicit physicians from different specialties and a range of practice settings. I also tried to interview doctors from a broad range of ages and ethnic groups. The snowball approach generated the entire sample and included the following: fourteen general internists, four cardiologists, two gastroenterologists, eleven family practitioners, seventeen geriatricians, and three critical care specialists. Practice settings included: seventeen in private or group practice, fourteen in community clinics, seven in public hospitals, four in university hospitals, two in community hospitals, two in health maintenance organizations, and five in nursing homes. The age range was thirty-two to seventy-one. There were twenty-one women and thirty men. In addition, the group included thirty-eight White, five Hispanic, three African American, and five Asian American physicians.

Interviews

An open-ended interview guide was constructed to elicit physician perspectives about decision making and responsibility in clinical medicine with elderly patients. The questions were intended to be relatively nondirective so that physicians could describe in their own words the dilemmas they face and the choices they make. Interviews elicited discussion of the following topics: description of current practice; problems and rewards in geriatric medicine; actual decision-making dilemmas; roles and responsibilities in treating the elderly who are frail and in the dying process; moral conflicts about the termination of life; relationships with family members; constraints on practice; and explanations of frailty and medical futility. Each interview was face-to-face and lasted approximately one hour. Interviews were audiotaped, and the tapes were later transcribed verbatim.

The physicians gave narrative accounts in response to my questions about difficult treatment decisions and the dilemmas they pose. They outlined the clinical problem and contextual features of at least one case (but often three or more), described the patient's problem(s) and their own response, emphasized the decision points and why those were troublesome, and, if the case had resolved, gave its final outcome. Their stories illustrate the uncertainty integral to much decision making in clinical medicine—not only in geriatrics—and the fact that the physicians may never know if they did the "right" thing.

NARRATIVES AND PHENOMENOLOGY

This chapter contributes to a phenomenology of clinical medicine[5] by exploring the definitions and meanings of patient-care dilemmas as physicians both construct and attempt to solve them in their narrative tellings. Phenomenologically, narratives work in at least two ways. First, their everyday discourse reveals naturally occurring concerns, meanings, and actions (Benner 1994). Narratives illustrate ways in which the storyteller remembers, engages, and anticipates both the problem and the relationship with the patient. The accounts reveal what concerns the storyteller—morally, medically, and practically—and illustrate how those aspects of concern cannot be disentangled. When physicians are given the opportunity to describe in detail their own subjective experience vis-à-vis patient care and concern, their narrative explanations—although constructed in response to an anthropologist's request—are presented as self-evident, spontaneous, and taken for granted. Full of language signifying emotion and values, they reveal how clinical dilemmas actually are understood and lived. The language of these narratives is a language of feelings at least as much as it is a language of rational deliberation.

Second, narratives illuminate features of the cultural and structural background to individual moral thought, feeling, and reflection. Narratives are built from shared but implicit understandings of the cultural world, problems, reasoning, and what works. Those understandings are the scaffolding on which clinical-moral quandary and deliberation rest. The stories physicians told constitute and are embedded in particular, yet open, cultural fields (Gordon 1994). For example, the stories depict the world of contemporary American medical practice delivered in a large urban setting, where the full range of biotechnologies, intensive care, nursing care, and ancillary social services are considered necessary and useful and are available frequently to all patients regardless of age or socioeconomic status. They emerge from the existing structures of health care delivery: the acute care hospital in which technologies create the need for diagnostic testing and life-prolonging care; the multidisciplinary team that manages all aspects of life and works toward risk reduction; and the intricacies of payment in which intensive care for elderly people is government financed, but housekeeping, transportation, medication, and hearing aids are not. In addition, the narratives express and locate some perplexing ironies of geriatric medicine, a domain fraught with ambiguity about the distinction between "natural" old age and disease process, conflict about whether disease should be treated, and questions about the role of medicine in dictating behavioral change and in prolonging life (Kaufman 1994, 1995). Stories also reflect tensions and oppositions characteristic of Anglo-American society more generally: surveillance versus freedom; care versus neglect; and dependence versus self-reliance. Physician narratives are thus conceived as cultural documents. As dynamic texts, they push cultural boundaries through their questioning of existing ways of knowing and acting and through their creation of avenues of choice. In addition, they interpret what is desirable, permissible, acceptable, or morally questionable.

DILEMMAS: THE NATURE OF CLINICAL-MORAL REASONING

In the analysis of the data, five kinds of dilemmas stood out as most commonly articulated by the fifty-one physicians, and each is posed here as a question or set of related questions: (1) How much intervention or treatment should there be: whether to treat or leave alone, hospitalize, treat as an outpatient, employ invasive diagnostic tests, treat with surgery or with drugs, place in the intensive care unit, place in a nursing home, how much to spend on an intervention? (2) How aggressive should one be with technologies for prolonging life? (3) How should one proceed with treatment: when there are differences of opinion about how to proceed and when medical judgment differs from patient or family wishes; when there is confusion about the nature of the patient's wishes; when the patient wants one thing, the family wants another, and the physician feels caught in the middle; when physicians disagree with one another about kinds of treatment to employ? (4) What does one do when the patient wants to remain independent in the community but is failing, according to family or other health providers? (5) How can one be certain where the lines are drawn between comfort care and life prolongation, for example, or between comfort care and euthanasia? How does one implement comfort care?

Having created this organized list of dilemmas out of the "flow" of data, I wish to emphasize that, articulated in narratives, actual dilemmas rarely emerged as discrete entities in the physicians' accounts. I have isolated them here for analytic purposes, to highlight the range of problems physicians describe. In the interviews themselves, two or more of these types of dilemmas frequently converged in the description of a particular case scenario, illustrating the phenomenological impossibility of the physician coming to terms with any one of them as a separate entity in the course of actual decision making. Ethical theorists have tended to approach such questions as though they were perceived by practitioners to be discrete and isolated, but the dilemmas expressed by these physicians rarely were unidimensional.

The narratives that follow enable us to discern ways in which physicians understand problematic issues in the treatment of their patients. They reveal how dilemmas cluster, merge with, and compound one another in physicians' reasoning. The narratives illustrate that clinical problems are neither conceived nor addressed by isolating their component parts; rather, they show the irreducible nature of dilemmas. Perhaps most significantly for bioethics, the narratives illustrate the fundamental connectedness of *clinical* and *moral* reasoning in the decision-making process.

I have chosen nine narratives from the data[6] to illustrate a range of long-term care problems that frequently confront practitioners who treat older patients. I have arranged them in three topical sets to reflect what I perceive to be a multidimensional chain or web of dilemmas in the phenomenology of geriatric medicine, rather than a discrete problem list. And I have placed them in groups of three to highlight variation in physicians' conceptualizations of certain themes.

The overarching clinical problem expressed by the fifty-one doctors, *degrees and means of intervention,* dominates all the chosen narratives and, in fact, most of the data collected. That problem is rooted in medicine's well-known and often-criticized directive—do something rather than nothing. The activist stance is shown here to be deeply troubling for practitioners in a broad range of circumstances. In the contexts of a growing elderly population, burgeoning chronic illness, and an overwhelming commitment to using technology, that fundamental directive, an essential feature of medicine's identity, has become a matter of profound ethical concern. The examples and discussion below contribute to the specification of the problem.

I begin with the broadly conceived issue of autonomy. The first set of narratives (Examples 1, 2, 3) illustrates a cultural conflict—permeating

American society beyond the boundaries of medicine—between safety and risk reduction, on the one hand, and freedom and independence, on the other. That conflict finds expression in the clinical dilemma: How much should and can one intervene? In the next set of cases that question becomes compounded with another: How aggressive should treatment be? Examples 4, 5, and 6 in the second set ponder issues of choice and responsibility in medicine in the face of the technological imperative. The last set of narratives joins the following additional questions to those posed by the others: What is comfort care? How does one provide it? And how can one reconcile comfort care with aggressive treatment?

How Much Should and Can One Intervene? Safety, Risk, and Surveillance

EXAMPLE 1

There is a guy who is about 78 or so who clearly has dementia and has had a couple of CVAs [strokes] and lives with his wife who is probably schizophrenic, psychotic to some degree. Their house is a disaster zone and the wife is housebound and she's just as obnoxious as she can be. This is one of the home care patients. The resident goes into this home and there are clothes everywhere and it smells of urine. There is not a big roach or rat history, but there is clutter and it's messy.

The resident, the case manager, and probably even Adult Protective Services are involved in this case. They all want to place this guy in [the county nursing home]. They are all saying, "He's in danger because his wife is so nuts, the house is a mess, and his quality of life is terrible." And I don't think he should be placed. My gut feeling is that they'd probably lived in a messy house even before he became ill. The evidence we have is that while the wife is nuts, she's also very committed to him. She tied a string around his waist, which is not an uncommon thing, it's a folk remedy. There are plenty of other patients who come in with strings around their waists. Probably she doesn't feed him right; that's the other thing. It brings up the issue of what do you do with people who have dementia but who are very clear, consistently, about their choice?

This guy does not want to be admitted to [a skilled nursing facility]. And there is a marginal living situation. I have spent hours and hours talking to people about this case. I feel like I really want to argue and advocate for him. It represents a class of problems you see in eldercare: older people who live in what are clearly less than ideal circumstances, who tolerate it fairly well, who aren't a danger to themselves. But it's really uncomfortable for us. You walk into somebody's house and it's disgusting. It's dirty and smelly and you say, "Get them out of there!"

So how much do we impose our values? We don't have access to the homes of younger people in the same way that we have access to the homes of the elderly. I suspect there are lots of people who live like this. If you live like this when you are young, why shouldn't you be able to live like this when you're old? It's a very tough one. . . . I don't know what will happen. We're trying to reframe the goals. One goal may be to have an agency come in and get the house cleaned up. That might be all that's required. (Geriatrician, hospital based)

EXAMPLE 2

An eighty-nine-year-old woman came in with a hip fracture. All she cared about was going home. She was mildly demented, not able to manage her money but coherent in terms of other sorts of decision making. There are examples of people in her category that come up all the time: not quite 100 percent competent, a little fuzzy around things like judgment and organizing their finances but not so incompetent as to be diagnosed by a psychiatrist. They're really in a gray area in terms of their ability to care for themselves, really on the borderline. For these kinds of people, it's hard to get services together. They want their independence. They won't sign over their finances to someone else, and they won't or can't pay for caregivers.

This particular woman lived up a flight of stairs, but she was very clear that she wanted to go home. The nursing staff said, "You can't send this woman home." And I said, "I sure can. We can worry about her safety, we can advise her, but it's her decision." And she was not worried very much about the stairs; she went home and did it. (Geriatrician, community clinic)

EXAMPLE 3

I had a patient that I really wasn't taking care of that long; I inherited her from one of the other doctors in this office because he didn't want to make house calls anymore. She was ninety-eight or ninety-nine years old and she lived with her daughter. They shared an apartment and the old lady could not leave the apartment because she had broken her hip. It's one of those places where she had to go up two flights of stairs. There was no elevator in the apartment house so she couldn't get up and down.

It was an unusual pair because the mother was alert and with it but physically very frail. The daughter, who was then in her early seventies, was demented. In fact I can still remember the mother taking me aside and saying, "I think my daughter has Alzheimer's disease." And that's exactly what happened. But the two of them managed together because the mother could still remember things and she would make lists and the daughter could still go out and shop if she had a list. I took care of the mother but not the daughter.

One day the daughter fell and broke her hip and ended up in the hospital. The social worker at the hospital, with the family, decided that the best solution was to put both of them in a nursing home. They put both of them in there. The daughter didn't really understand what was going on. She still keeps asking me when she is going home. I don't know what they did with the dog. The mother had been doing just fine at home. Nothing had happened to her. She only survived about four months in the nursing home. And the daughter was totally confused and wandered around and had to be tied in a chair so "she wouldn't hurt herself." She was no longer ambulatory.

There's no reason why they should have been moved out of their apartment. They were both ambulatory enough to get around the apartment. They were both safe in the apartment and the old lady was alert enough to call for help on the phone. All they needed was to have somebody come in and do the cooking and the cleaning. I'm sure that shortened the old lady's life. And the daughter has been sort of chronically depressed and unhappy because her mother was the only person she identified with and now she's gone. She won't take any medicine.

It was sort of a disaster. It was a complicated situation because they were two patients with two different doctors. But the family, nieces and nephews, were interested in both old ladies being placed where they could be cared for so nobody would have to bother with them. But, you know, that's very frustrating. I don't know what I could have done. It was not my decision. I just got the phone call from the nursing home saying, "We now have your patient and the daughter is here also and the daughter doesn't want to be in the nursing home. Would you see about that?" (Internist, private practice)

A language of risk, need, safety, and surveillance has emerged in the United States in the last decade or so as a cultural response to the "growing problem" of old people in America. Recent attention to risk and the elderly may result from the fact that risk is on the rise as a cultural category (Douglas and Wildavsky 1982). The language of risk has become a framework for understanding the perils of the Western industrial world (Clark 1984). It has been said that we live in a "risk society" (Beck 1992), a world made dangerous by technologies of war and industry. Much understanding of what constitutes danger, some criteria for decision making, and some public policies are based on questions of risk assessment, avoidance, and acceptance in everyday life. Public consciousness of risk and its reverberations in all areas of life has perhaps never been higher (Nelkin 1989; Slovic 1987).

Risk awareness as both a function and an expression of medicine is now firmly embedded in understanding the role of medical care in late-twentieth-century U.S. society. In geriatrics, much activity in the medical care of old people concerns the biomedically framed "need" to assess and minimize the risks to which both health professionals and the broader public feel older people are exposed, or that their functionally limited bodies, selves, and lives apparently embody. The elderly are considered *at risk* for falls, institutionalization, physical and mental decline, and are considered *in need* of age-appropriate medical assessments, special services, and case management (Dill 1993; Kaufman and Becker 1995). *Surveillance* of their hygiene, finances, abilities, activities, and associates therefore is justified as medically, socially, and morally appropriate.

For frail elderly in American society, there exists a seemingly permanent tension between safety and supervision, on the one hand, and risk and independence, on the other. The need to reduce risk competes with the all-pervasive value of autonomy, the right to freely choose, have options, and be left alone. These values clash in the delivery of health care to create ethical conflict for physicians as they attempt to care for their frail patients in the community. Physicians' solutions to that conflict are both individual, reflecting their feelings about independence and attitudes toward patient advocacy, and socially derived, reflecting pressures brought by family members and other professionals as well as by the institutions in which they work. Physicians 1 and 2 work in hospital and clinic settings well regarded for their attention to geriatric care, where teams of professionals "holistically" scrutinize the lives of their clients to treat and manage the whole person. Example 3 illustrates the poor fit between medical and social services (resulting, in large part, from Medicare policy) and the accompanying low priority placed on social and long-term health care services in the community by service providers and consumers.

Authority and responsibility vis-à-vis risk management are shown here to be contextual and variable. In narrative Examples 1 and 2, physician authority is negotiable: The narrators honored independence and enabled their patients to remain at home, at least for the time being. In Example 3, the physician described himself as powerless to solve the conflict between safety and independence as he would have preferred. Responsibility in all three cases was realized in advocacy for the patient's freedom to remain at home in spite of frailty, dementia, and other medical conditions. This particular manifestation of responsibility reflects that these physicians have chosen to practice geriatrics; they enjoy working with older people and feel a sense of duty toward them. Other physicians, especially those not trained in geriatrics, would respond differently.

How Aggressive Should One Be? The Pull of Technology

EXAMPLE 4

There are dilemmas regularly. I'll take the freshest one. Some guy came in last Friday after climbing the hill up to his house. He's seventy years old, high cholesterol, had chest pain, and really felt tired. Never had angina before. So, Friday the cardiogram was okay. First level of decision making: Was this pain so bad that the guy should go into the hospital with this first episode of angina? Should he be watched for a real potential, preinfarction syndrome? You know, cardiograms don't prove that he didn't have a heart attack. So I put him in the hospital until I know if his enzymes are negative and that the EKG [electrocardiogram] didn't miss it. So that was tough. I told him to go home, rest, take medicine to reduce the risk of angina. I called the lab Saturday morning to make sure his enzymes were negative, which they were, and Monday I arranged for him to do a treadmill test. He had the test, but he has bad ankles. So he only *sort of* did a treadmill test. He got to the percentage of exercise he was supposed to, but he wasn't in it for very long and he had minor changes in his cardiogram. But the changes didn't occur right away and he didn't have any symptoms.

So then what do you do? It's not like you're talking about a cold. You are talking about a guy who could drop dead, okay? I could have said right away, "He's got to get a better test," a $1200 test to see how bad his heart disease is. I'm certain he had angina. The question is, Is this an impending catastrophe or is he just going to have angina for a while? I mean, every adult in the United States who has angina shouldn't get that test. So I said to him, "Stay off the medicine. If you get pain, then you restart the medicine. If you still have pain, you've got to do the test." But I'm apprehensive because I just reviewed a case of a good doctor who had a person get a treadmill test and was told by the cardiologist that the test was normal. When looking back on it, it wasn't. And that patient did what I had my patient do. That guy was young and into racquetball and his doctor told him, "If you get more pain, call me up." And the guy went back and played racquetball and dropped dead. So, that case is real fresh in my mind. It's a difficult decision, how much testing I do. (Internist, private practice)

EXAMPLE 5

To me the most difficult decisions are those that involve someone who is so frail that it's difficult to know how aggressive to be for the treatment. It's also very difficult if it's a patient I'm not familiar with. A lot of things happen when the regular physician has the day off or it's a weekend and you have to jump in and evaluate someone that you don't know.

I took care of a woman in her nineties, very demented, with Parkinson's disease. I was told that when she heard that others had died she said, "Could they move over so I can lay down with them and die also?" She wasn't very happy about being alive in this state. She developed a fever and very low blood pressure and I was told that she did this occasionally and it was usually because of an upper respiratory infection. In this organization we will often take care of people who are pretty sick. We'll try and manage them for a few hours and see if they'll turn around with fluids and a lot of attention. But by the end of the day she was doing very poorly. I wondered what we should do because she was so sick and frail; maybe it was just best to keep her comfortable.

But not knowing her and not knowing how the family would feel, I admitted her to the hospital and I did everything I could do on the day of admission to make sure she would stay alive. I checked her blood for evidence of infection; I started her on antibiotics and gave her a lot of fluids so the blood pressure would come up, but she remained comatose. The next day I didn't really do much. She wasn't turning around. I made a decision not to look into what was wrong, figuring that if it was something that needed an operation, I didn't think she would be operated on. But I just didn't feel comfortable.

Another physician took over her case three days after she was hospitalized. Some information accumulated and that physician decided to progress further. In an abdominal ultrasound we found that there were gallstones despite the fact that the woman had had her gallbladder removed. There were some retained stones in her bile and some of the staff thought, "We wouldn't operate on her, but maybe we can do a relatively safe invasive procedure and try to get those stones out because then she might improve." That's not what I would have done. As it turned out, there were some stones removed and she was discharged from the hospital, but she expired the day she was discharged.

I felt that no matter what was done it wouldn't have helped because she was so malnourished and frail. But I have a lot of trouble with situations like that, not knowing how far to push when I'm really very confident the situation is dismal. How hard should I try to maintain someone's life when I think my intervention will only have the person last a few days longer? It's also difficult when you're working with a group of physicians and each physician might treat a case in a different way. . . . Sometimes it's very difficult to know when to stop being very aggressive because you get very attached to people. We care a lot about them and I can make the mistake of thinking that keeping them alive is good for them. When it may not be. (Geriatrician, community clinic)

EXAMPLE 6

I had a patient who was a very vigorous eighty-four- or eighty-five-year-old man who was living independently and was basically fairly healthy.

He had some chronic renal insufficiency and atrial fibrillation. He started getting angina and we debated whether or not we should treat him symptomatically, which we did. He came back a few weeks later with a myocardial infarction and was having angina on an increasing basis. So the decision was made to go ahead and do an angiogram. Through all of this, he was in agreement and his family was in agreement. We had discussed not doing heroic interventions for irreversible conditions. He had been clear on that. But at the same time, it was sort of like, "Well, maybe we should do just this much."

The angiogram showed in fact that he had fairly severe stenosis in a couple of vessels. He did okay through the angiogram but then about twelve hours later had a major stroke. . . . He was at increased risk for stroke anyway. It could have been that he was going to have a stroke anyway, but the association is always one that you worry about. That's one of the things that can happen when they've got the catheter in; they can loosen bits of grunge from inside the vessels. He ended up aphasic [without speech], which for this man was just about the worst thing that could have happened because he was a very verbal, intelligent man. It was something very hard for him to deal with.

We sort of went in with the idea of trying to get some rehabilitation going. You know, forgetting about the idea of a bad heart. He just had a series of one thing after another going wrong. He went from the hospital to a rehab facility then back to the hospital and then to a nursing home. It became clear that we really weren't going to be able to get him back on his feet again. And ultimately, after about two months, we came to the conclusion, with him and his daughter, that we weren't going to be doing anything more. We went for comfort care and he died in the nursing home.

With 20/20 hindsight, if I had known at the beginning what was going to happen, then of course the decisions would have been quite different. It's sort of an ongoing process where you're deciding at some point that you've done more than you can or as much as you can and its time to call it quits.

I had the feeling that he wanted to call it quits a good month sooner than his daughter did. He was clearly deteriorating. There was clearly a point at which we could stop doing things or we could keep doing things, but it wasn't a decision that had to be made immediately. I could continue to kind of work on keeping things going for a week or two to give his daughter a chance to adjust to the idea that he wasn't going to get better. And so in this case, I was willing to kind of go with the daughter. Also, I had the feeling that there was still a potential that we could turn things around again and go on. I tend to be very optimistic about that and I may be pushing a little harder than the patient would want me to, but I figure in terms of keeping someone alive for another week if they are going to be dying slowly, another week is not going to make that much difference in the long run. (Geriatrician, private practice)

The questions of whether to employ or forego invasive diagnostic tests or aggressive treatment procedures and how much to do loom large in these three cases. There are no clear-cut formulas physicians can use for arriving at solutions, yet the press to do something that will move toward more precise diagnosis or cure usually outweighs other options. It is extremely difficult, as these narratives illustrate, for physicians to forge a middle path of employing some, but not all, relevant interventions and still "feel comfortable." The technological imperative in medicine—to order ever more diagnostic tests, to perform procedures, to intervene with respirators and feeding tubes to prolong life or stave off death—is an important variable in contemporary medical practice. It is a discourse that determines thought and action, and it provides a restrictive language—of "do everything," "not very much," and "only a little"— through which choices are framed and dilemmas are understood. By confining choice to black-and-white terms and by forcing physicians to conceive of good, adequate, appropriate care as embodied in maximum intervention, the technological imperative narrows doctors' field of possibilities and thus removes moral options. The impact of the technological imperative is especially destabilizing to moral sensibility when the patient is very old and has multiple, complex medical problems.

The available divergent choices compete for dominance as physicians sometimes struggle to resolve a case and bring a sense of closure to the narrative: Does one need to know precisely what the clinical picture is by getting the most thorough diagnostic test available, or does one reject the test in favor of keeping the patient's costs down and sparing him or her perhaps needless discomfort, suffering, or iatrogenic illness? Should one attempt to cure the acute problems of a demented, frail, and very old patient, or should one decide against those options and possibly shorten (or actually not prolong) her life by days, weeks, or maybe even months, in favor of making her as comfortable as possible?

Physicians face profound dilemmas when they "don't feel comfortable" either ordering invasive procedures for old and frail individuals (as in Example 5) or deciding not to order the most expensive, thorough diagnostic tests (Example 4). Narratives 5 and 6 show how discomfort cries for some kind of clinical-moral resolution because the dilemmas encompass tensions between personal and medical values about action to extend life and cause or prolong suffering. Physician 5 noted her personal preference for wanting to forego invasive treatment because of the frailty and advanced age of the patient: Any procedure she ordered would add to the patient's pain. Yet she was distressed knowing her opinion differed from that of other physicians. Her fundamental confusion and uncertainty both about medicine's uses of aggressive treatment to "keep them alive" and her own responsibility in "situations like that" are powerfully expressed in the last lines of the narrative. Physician 6 said, "Well, maybe we should do just this much" when faced with the patient who was "having angina on an increasing basis." In that case, an intervention conceived to be mid-way between the extremes of being "heroic" and doing nothing—the only "good" compromise available in the interventionist discourse—was the morally preferable choice although it had a disastrous clinical outcome.

Responsible medicine has been defined in the contemporary era by action and continued treatment to the point of cure, stability of the condition, or death of the patient. Only when outcomes are repeatedly negative and the patient has an obviously downward course, as in Example 6 (in which an angiogram potentially caused a stroke), does the option of "calling it quits" or "not doing much" emerge as viable. In its ideal conception, responsibility in medicine is conceived *through* action. But physicians struggle with that ideal as they confront multiple decision points and search for morally acceptable treatments and actions. As these cases illustrate, the path chosen may emerge as the "right" decision, clinically and morally, only after the case is closed with the patient's recovery, stabilization, or death. But tension between the clinical and moral may emerge as well: Physician 4 felt socially and economically responsible when he chose not to order an expensive diagnostic test, but he worried about the clinical ramifications of his decision. Regardless of which decision the physician makes, knowledge that the other possible choice in this black-and-white world would have been better can remain to haunt the physician as can a nagging sense of existing, yet unarticulated options. Those other possibilities can inhibit or prevent a sense of narrative closure and moral resolution.

The Nature of Comfort Care and Its Reconciliation with Aggressive Treatment: The Blurring of Boundaries

EXAMPLE 7

In caring for frail and demented old patients, the primary goal is comfort. Sometimes that's best addressed by simply treating symptoms. On the other hand, sometimes it's much more efficient to make people comfortable by making a diagnosis and treating something specifically. So it doesn't just mean symptomatic care. But I think that's the major goal and I think pro-longation of life is certainly secondary.

Sometimes with demented people it's hard to tell whether they're suffering or not, and if so, what they're suffering from. But we try to relieve suffering to the extent that it's possible. But a typical situation here is that a demented person in a nursing home can't swallow very well, food goes down his lungs, he gets pneumonia, the people in the nursing home panic, they send the patient to the hospital, the doctor panics, the patient goes to the intensive care unit, and the whole sequence of events and interventions gets played out.

I might have a lot of judgments about the demented person with pneumonia who comes in from the nursing home. This person shouldn't be in the intensive care unit, shouldn't be in the hospital, probably should be back at the nursing home, probably should be allowed to die. But he is the person who is in the intensive care unit and you are stuck with him. So the best thing, the most efficient thing to do is to try and get him well as quick as possible so you can reverse the process and get him going back to the nursing home. So what that means is doing a certain amount of aggressive or active work. Instead of withdrawing, you might actually think, "Well, the quickest way out of this is to get him over these little humps so then I can get him out of here." So it gets tricky sometimes. (Critical care specialist, hospital based)

EXAMPLE 8

There is a man with bad peripheral vascular disease and in essence has a foot that is completely cold and has no circulation. He has had several strokes. He was depressed and saying, "Let me go; I don't want all this stuff done." And the family members, his children, were in agreement. He had been given the option of hospice-type care. Then a new acute problem developed and so now we've got to take care of it. We can't let this sit because it's causing him a lot of pain and discomfort. Pain relief is needed and we've got to do something. It's either keep him comfortable and let him die of a gangrenous foot, take the foot off, or try and do something else.

What we ended up doing was a kind of bypass, which means we turned under the skin and grafted all the way down the leg, which fortunately for him worked—at least for the time being. Those types tend to close up within a year, but at least for the time being he's out of pain. It wasn't a major intervention. But you know, you can't always come up with stuff like that. (Geriatrician, private practice)

EXAMPLE 9

A woman with dementia who begins to fail rapidly starts refusing to eat—almost growls at you—then has a stroke and cancer. Then the sister says, "She didn't want any artificial feeding through IVs [intravenous lines]." So you'd think that makes it easy. Wrong. Because then you come in on a different level. And you are conflicted about whether you can just do a little bit, whether you can let somebody die of thirst. They're not thirsty. It's not uncomfortable. But they die of dehydration. And then you can say, "Sure, that was the patient's wishes." These days, none of this paternalism—The doctor knows what's best for you.

I could keep her alive with an IV. It's me. It's the doctor. Before she was so sick with the stroke and the cancer, she was refusing food. I could say, "I think we ought to give her a little IV, and make her a little more comfortable, and let's just see what happens." It's very hard at times to resist doing something that would keep somebody alive a little longer. That's difficult.

In this case, I didn't give her an IV, but I didn't like it. So I did all these other little things to justify it. I scolded the nurses for not giving her better mouth care; I wanted her turned [to prevent pressure sores] and kept comfortable. And then when she was infected, I gave her some antibiotics, which is almost incongruous, you know. But I didn't want her to have these germs multiplying within her. It didn't sound aesthetic to me. So it's little things. You do it for yourself, some of these things, to be perfectly honest.

You know, it could have gone either way and obviously I was conflicted as to which way to go with this one. So many times I was tempted to give her a little fluid. It would make me feel better. And I had to fight that too. But we do make these arbitrary decisions. We have to cope with these decisions every day. (Geriatrician, skilled nursing facility)

The dominant vocabulary available to American doctors to know and realize their options when a patient's death appears near is both thin and decidedly oppositional: comfort versus heroics; symptomatic care or aggressive treatment; withdrawing or acting; "keep him comfortable and let him die" or "try and do something" (as in Example 8). That language, produced in the wake of the technological imperative described above, constitutes and delimits the nature of *good* practice vis-à-vis death and denies the possibility of other narrative understandings of both what to do and how to be (Gordon 1994; May 1994). Reasoning and decision making become narrowly focused and constrained.

As the language of risk has shaped medical understanding of old people's bodies and lives and framed many goals of geriatric medicine (Kaufman 1994), so has the oppositional vocabulary of medical choice framed ethical practice when confronting the dying process. One fights death by acting "heroically" or one gives up, "fails": "We have nothing more to offer"; "There is nothing more we can do." The technological imperative made fighting death logical, routine, good, and important. "Comfort" and "withdrawal" became euphemisms for the essential fact that treatment had failed. Although this discourse remains pervasive and powerful (SUPPORT Principal Investigators 1995), the desire for an alternative to this oppositional vocabulary, expressed in the last decade or so by both practitioners and patients along with their families, produced "palliative care" or "comfort care" (Institute of Medicine 1997), an ethical practice that focuses on reducing pain and assisting or easing respiration, with the best drugs and technologies available while not interfering in the body's natural dying process. Palliative care is defined as purposeful action. It, too, can be aggressive—"There is a great deal the physician can do." It has been produced socially to "fit" medicine's deeply rooted directive of "doing something," even when death is expected.

The physicians in this study spoke *in the abstract* of the importance of palliative or comfort care for very old people and how, at the end of life, the correct moral choice was always the comfort of the patient rather than high technology heroics to prolong life. Yet as they described particular cases in response to my questions and probes, it became evident that the line between comfort care and aggressive medical intervention that would delay death was not clear *in practice* in many instances. The confusion over what actually constitutes palliation, whether that set of practices can be separated from unnecessary, optional, or unwanted life-prolonging interventions, patients' lack of clarity about whether they want life prolongation or "comfort," and the sometimes questionable moment in which comfort care merges with euthanasia all were sources of dilemmas for physicians.

Most physicians in this study said that the ideal role of the physician in the care of the frail or demented elderly was to provide comfort. But some of them noted that the physician must assess *how* to provide comfort and that diagnosing disease and treating acute problems, even when that requires the use of invasive procedures, may be the best way to achieve that goal. Thus palliative or comfort care is not really a discrete activity, identifiable in the abstract. It is defined by physicians *in relation* to kinds and degrees of treatment. As one informant noted, "Commonly, we end up in situations where a frail person comes in with five problems at once. They don't want too much workup, but they want some comfort for their pain or their discomfort and you don't know how to treat it without working it up. There are constant judgments like that" (geriatrician, community clinic).

So comfort care is an ambiguous notion. The dilemma of how much to intervene in attempting to reach the goal of comfort is raised by the doctors as an open and everpresent question. Physician 7 emphasized that medicine is focused largely on and driven by the solving of acute problems with the most technology available. Therefore "comfort" has to be redefined continually in the context of an action-oriented health care delivery system. In this scenario, aggressive acute care intervention is rationalized as the immediate, most efficient means to enable the patient to later receive palliation only. That rationale arises in response to the realities of high technology medicine imposed on one physician's values. It emerges because a single practitioner can never make decisions in a vacuum. Each physician is dependent on the existence of other practitioners' judgments and actions. The push toward hospitalization and using technology provides the context, in Example 7 as well as many others, for assigning priority to aggressive acute treatment, even when "allowing" the patient to die is the ultimate goal. That physician's description provides a good example of how one practitioner's ideals must be continually negotiated amidst pressures from institutional forces.

Example 8 shows how the importance of aggressive treatment for an acute condition causing pain takes precedence over some abstract notion of comfort, even in situations where patient, family, and doctor agree that hospice or terminal care is preferable. That physician was able to implement a temporary form of pain relief that was not as invasive as amputation, but she noted that physicians cannot always create or invoke compromise treatments, that is, solutions that satisfy the patient's desire for minimal intervention and, at the same time, allow the practitioner to alleviate an acute medical problem.

Physician 9 did not see artificial nutrition and hydration as a means to comfort care, but another doctor might have. Rather, his conflict was over whether to provide fluids so that he could be sure that the patient would not die of dehydration. But he held back and honored the patient's and family's wishes for no food and fluids. Yet his personal values dictated that he *do* something. He chose to intervene by giving antibiotics for an infection and by rigorously insisting that the patient be given "comfort" in the form of attention to her oral hygiene and bed sore prevention. Comfort care was defined and implemented in that case by the physician's personal values in tension with patient and family wishes.

The clinical reasoning revealed in these three narratives, and in others, suggests that in their actual work physicians often cannot describe the boundaries between comfort care and fighting death. Although the vocabulary creates discrete categories of knowledge and the two theoretical options that constitute good practice, the words do not actually designate separate phenomena. Both palliation and intervention are *defined and negotiated* for each patient in local contexts of institutional pressures, patient and family demands, and the physician's personal values.

NARRATIVE, CULTURE, ETHICS

American bioethics has focused its attention on moral quandaries that occur in medical settings and has offered prescriptive guides for their potential solutions. It generally addresses well-articulated dilemmas about decision making and overlooks issues not specifically identified as morally problematic or clinically derived (Fox 1991; Gordon 1994). This chapter has explored only the acknowledged and circumscribed subject of bioethics: clinical-moral dilemmas as they are explicitly framed in the medical arena. Within this particular conception of the moral–medical relationship, an ethnographic approach has been employed to expand conceptions of ethical concern and practice and to uncover relationships between "ethical" and "cultural" knowledge and experience.

In analyzing narratives from fifty-one physicians, at least three dimensions of the phenomenology of clinical medicine are evident. First, dilemmas emerge from the flow of everyday subjective experience embedded in a structural and cultural context, and they are not isolated, cannot be isolated, into component parts for deliberation. Instead, dilemmas are revealed to be clusters or multidimensional webs of tough problems about doing the right thing. And they emerge from language that invokes tensions about risk reduction and independence, the high value placed on technology use and action, and the social, economic, and political pressures imposed on delivering care in various institutional settings.

Second, clinical knowledge is shown to be inextricably tied to moral knowledge about the patient, who is himself conceived in a sociocultural context. Resolving a problem means knowing what is "good for" the patient (Mattingly 1993; Smith and Churchill 1986) and then acting on that knowledge. In many instances, as we have seen, doctors admit to not knowing what is *good* for the patient. That lack of clarity is grounded in their not knowing what is *good* in the science and practice of medicine (Smith and Churchill 1986:43–44).

Third, the clinical-moral dilemmas these doctors formulated—how much to intervene to reduce risk, how aggressive to be, and how "comfort" and "treatment" can be reconciled—point to the often-murky relationship of dilemmas to the goals of medicine. An individual practitioner may have clear-cut treatment goals and know what is right and good for a particular patient, only to have those goals derailed or reinterpreted by a health care delivery system focused on safety and risk reduction and committed to using advanced technology, or by patients and families who demand that everything or nothing be done. Or competing goals may vie for dominance in a specific situation, as in cases of whether to hospitalize a patient, place a patient in a nursing home, order invasive and painful tests, perform surgery, and begin artificial feeding. Sometimes physicians do not have well-defined goals, as narrative 5 poignantly illustrates, especially about justification for prolonging a frail life. The relationship of goals to individual practitioner responsibility often is fraught with ambiguity and, at times, with anguish and frustration.

Phenomenologically, these physician narratives speak to an essential lack of clarity about the doctor's role and identity vis-à-vis medical goals (Brody 1992). In addition, the narratives speak to broader connections between culture and ethics. Their personal meaningfulness, emotional salience, and cultural constitution show that ethical practice is neither based on abstract rationality nor applied to actual problems from some neutral position. Rather, the stories describe a grounded ethics, a reality of unfolding clinical-moral experience embedded in the particular structural conditions and cultural-medical discourses of geriatric medicine and late-twentieth-century American preoccupations with risk, technology, and the avoidance of death. We have seen how those conditions and discourses create specific kinds of moral quandary and prescribe definite avenues of ethical action for their solution. The narratives also reveal how those forces shape knowledge about how one ought to be a physician, what actions are right or wrong, and how one creates and defines values in everyday practice.

Narratives offer exemplars of ways of knowing how to act and how to *be* a doctor. Yet their individuality and particularity are not merely personal. Narratives are cultural documents, cultural representations reflecting shared understandings of language and institutions. They illustrate structures of power and knowledge and reflect crises and impasses in the "ethics of the social body" (Kleinman 1995). They describe a "truth" whose features are publicly known. The normative relevance of narratives lies not in a foundation of moral principles but rather in the deeply embedded and shared nature of the stories themselves, that they are constituted through multiple cultural worlds. The categories of risk, surveillance, control, and action; the embodiment of "the good" in both the technological imperative and the vocabulary of heroism versus comfort; the ambiguous stance of geriatric medicine toward death; and the structural frameworks through which contemporary health care is delivered[7] provide the norms, the basis of both "cultural" and "ethical" understanding.

This chapter has contributed to a phenomenology of clinical medicine and an ethnography of ethical knowledge and practice in geriatrics. It is hoped that a growing ethnographic literature on clinical dilemmas per se as well as on other forms of ethical understanding and comportment can expand perspectives and understandings of the relationship between culture and ethics and thus forge a more fulfilling dialogue between ethicists and social scientists.

Notes

Acknowledgments: The research for this chapter was supported by National Institute on Aging grant AG11538 (Sharon R. Kaufman, Principal Investigator). I am indebted to the physicians who participated in this project. I thank all the conference participants, and especially Barry Hoffmaster, for their insights and comments on earlier drafts.

1. This conception is drawn from the work of Cheryl Mattingly (1991, 1993, 1998).

2. The stories of patient care are subjective accounts, self-evident and taken for granted by their authors. They are bracketed as stories from the flow of everyday experience.

3. "Physician Dilemmas in Geriatric Care," National Institute on Aging, grant AG11538.

4. Much of geriatric medical practice, as reported by physicians in this study, is routine and not morally problematic. The interviews sought the reporting of dilemmas. The narratives are not intended to represent geriatric medicine. Rather, they focus on one feature of it: interactions and events conceived as clinical-moral problems.

5. The term "phenomenological" has been used increasingly in the social sciences to refer to perspectives that are concerned with the natives' point of view, with meaning, subjectivity, or consciousness—perspectives that account for

"the phenomenon" under investigation as irreducible and autonomous in its own right. Anthropologists and sociologists have used the term to refer to both "a manner or style of thinking" about the nature of subjective experience (Merleau-Ponty 1962 [1945]) and a method that brackets, to the extent possible, the investigator's categories of meaning (Frank 1986; Watson and Watson-Franke 1985). The clinical narratives here are reflections of past events, yet they are "given" and presented as self-evident.

6. More than 100 narrative case examples were reported by the fifty-one physicians during interviews.

7. Structural frameworks include the following: Medicare and Medicaid policies, managed care, critical care, long-term care, and fragmented fee for service.

REFERENCES

Anspach, Renee R. 1993. *Deciding Who Lives*. Berkeley: University of California Press.

Beck, U. 1992. *Risk Society*. Beverly Hills, CA: Sage.

Benner, Patricia. 1994. The Tradition and Skill of Interpretive Phenomenology in Studying Health, Illness, and Caring Practices. In *Interpretive Phenomenology*, ed. Patricia Benner, 99–128. Thousand Oaks, CA: Sage.

Bosk, Charles. 1979. *Forgive and Remember*. Chicago: University of Chicago Press.

———. 1992. *All God's Mistakes: Genetic Counseling in a Pediatric Hospital*. Chicago: University of Chicago Press.

Brody, Howard. 1992. *The Healer's Power*. New Haven, CT: Yale University Press.

Clark, Jack A., Deborah A. Potter, and John B. McKinlay. 1991. Bringing Social Structure Back into Clinical Decision Making. *Social Science and Medicine* 32:853–866.

Clark, Margaret. 1984. The Cultural Patterning of Risk Seeking Behavior. *UCSF Mobius* 4:97–107.

Dill, Ann. 1993. Defining Needs, Defining Systems: A Critical Analysis. *Gerontologist* 33:453–460.

Douglas, Mary, and Aaron Wildavsky. 1982. *Risk and Culture*. Berkeley: University of California Press.

Fox, Renee C. 1991. The Evolution of American Bioethics: A Sociological Perspective. In *Social Science Perspectives on Medical Ethics*, ed. George Weisz, 201–220. Philadelphia: University of Pennsylvania Press.

Fox, Renee C., and Judith P. Swazey. 1992. *Spare Parts*. New York: Oxford University Press.

Frank, Arthur. 1995. *The Wounded Storyteller*. Chicago: University of Chicago Press.

Frank, Gelya. 1986. On Embodiment: A Case Study of Congenital Limb Deficiency in American Culture. *Culture, Medicine and Psychiatry* 10:189–219.

Good, Byron. 1994. *Medicine, Rationality, and Experience*. New York: Cambridge University Press.

Good, Mary-Jo Del Vecchio, Byron J. Good, Cynthia Schaffer, and Stuart E. Lind. 1990. American Oncology and the Discourse on Hope. *Culture, Medicine, and Psychiatry* 14:59–79.

Good, Mary-Jo DelVecchio, Tseunetsugo Munakata, Yasuki Kobayashi, Cheryl Mattingly, and Byron J. Good. 1994. Oncology and Narrative Time. *Social Science and Medicine* 38:855–862.

Gordon, Deborah R. 1990. Embodying Illness, Embodying Cancer. *Culture, Medicine and Psychiatry* 14:275–297.

———. 1994. The Ethics of Ambiguity and Concealment around Cancer. In *Interpretive Phenomenology*, ed. Patricia Benner, 279–317. Thousand Oaks, CA: Sage.

Hoffmaster, Barry. 1992. Can Ethnography Save the Life of Medical Ethics? *Social Science and Medicine* 35:1421–1431.

———. 1994. The Forms and Limits of Medical Ethics. *Social Science and Medicine* 39:1155–1164.

Hunter, Kathryn Montgomery. 1991. *Doctors' Stories: The Narrative Structure of Medical Knowledge*. Princeton, NJ: Princeton University Press.

Institute of Medicine. 1997. *Approaching Death: Improving Care at the End of Life*. Washington, DC: National Academy Press.

Kaufman, Sharon R., 1993. *The Healer's Tale: Transforming Medicine and Culture*. Madison: University of Wisconsin Press.

———. 1994. Old Age, Disease, and the Discourse on Risk. *Medical Anthropology Quarterly* 9:76–93.

———. 1995. Decision Making, Responsibility, and Advocacy in Geriatric Medicine. *Gerontologist* 35:481–488.

Kaufman, Sharon R., and Gay Becker. 1995. Frailty, Risk, and Choice: Cultural Discourses and the Question of Responsibility. In *Older Adults' Decision-making and the Law*, ed. Michael Smyer, K. Warner Schaie, and Marshall Kapp, 48–69. New York: Springer.

Kleinman, Arthur. 1988. *The Illness Narratives*. New York: Basic Books.

———. 1995. Anthropology of Medicine. In *Encyclopedia of Bioethics*, revised ed., ed. Warren T. Reich. New York: Simon and Schuster Macmillan.

Kleinman, Arthur, and Joan Kleinman. 1991. Suffering and Its Professional Transformation: Toward an Ethnography of Interpersonal Experience. *Culture, Medicine, and Psychiatry* 15:275–301.

Koenig, Barbara. 1988. The Technological Imperative in Medical Practice: The Social Creation of a "Routine" Treatment. In *Biomedicine Examined*, eds. Margaret Lock and Deborah Gordon, 465–496. Dordrecht: Kluwer.

———. 1993. Cultural Diversity in Decision-Making about Care at the End of Life. Institute of Medicine Workshop: Dying, Decisionmaking, and Appropriate Care. Washington, DC: Institute of Medicine.

Lindenbaum, Shirley, and Margaret Lock, eds. 1993. *Knowledge, Power and Practice: The Anthropology of Medicine and Everyday Life*. Berkeley: University of California Press.

Marshall, Patricia A. 1992. Anthropology and Bioethics. *Medical Anthropology Quarterly* 6:49–73.

Mattingly, Cheryl. 1991. The Narrative Nature of Clinical Reasoning. *American Journal of Occupational Therapy* 45:998–1005.

———. 1993. What Is "the Good" for This Patient? Paper presented at the annual meeting of the *American Anthropological Association.* Washington, DC, November 17–21.

———. 1994. The Concept of Therapeutic "Emplotment." *Social Science and Medicine* 38:811–822.

———. 1998. *Healing Dramas and Clinical Plots.* Cambridge: Cambridge University Press.

May, William F. 1994. The Virtues in a Professional Setting. In *Medicine and Moral Reasoning,* eds. K. W. M. Fulford, Grant R. Gilleltt, and Janet Martin Soskice, 75–90. New York: Cambridge University Press.

Merleau-Ponty, Maurice. 1962. *Phenomenology of Perception,* trans. Colin Smith, London: Routledge and Kegan Paul. Originally published as Phénoménologie de la Perception (Paris: Editions Gallimard, 1945).

Mishler, Elliot. 1984. *The Discourse of Interviews: Dialectics of Medical Interviews.* Norwood, NJ: Ablex.

Muller, Jessica H. 1992. Shades of Blue: The Negotiation of Limited Codes by Medical Residents. *Social Science and Medicine* 34:885–898.

———. 1994. Anthropology, Bioethics, and Medicine: A Provocative Trilogy. *Medical Anthropology Quarterly* 8:448–467.

Muller, Jessica H., and Barbara Koenig. 1988. On the Boundary of Life and Death: The Definition of Dying by Medical Residents. In *Biomedicine Examined,* eds. Margaret Lock and Deborah Gordon, 351–376. Dordrecht: Kluwer.

Nelkin, Dorothy. 1989. Communicating Technological Risk. *American Review of Public Health* 10:95–113.

Pellegrino, Edmund D. 1994. The Four Principles and the Doctor-Patient Relationship. In *Principles of Health Care Ethics,* ed. R. Gillon, 353–366. Chichester, U.K.: Wiley.

Rhodes, Lorna A. 1993. The Shape of Action: Practice in Public Psychiatry. In *Knowledge, Power and Practice,* eds. Shirley Lindenbaum and Margaret Lock, 129–146. Berkeley: University California Press.

Slovic, Paul. 1987. Perception of Risk. *Science* 236:280–285.

Smith, Harmon L., and Larry R. Churchill. 1986. *Professional Ethics and Primary Care Medicine.* Durham, NC: Duke University Press.

SUPPORT Principal Investigators. 1995. A Controlled Trial to Improve Care for Seriously Ill Hospitalized Patients. *JAMA* 274:1591–1634.

Taylor, Kathryn M. 1988. Physicians and the Disclosure of Undesirable Information. In *Biomedicine Examined,* eds. Margaret Lock and Deborah Gordon, 441–464. Dordrecht: Kluwer.

Waitzkin, Howard. 1991. *The Politics of Medical Encounters.* New Haven, CT: Yale University Press.

Watson, Lawrence C., and Maria-Barbara Watson-Franke. 1985. *Interpreting Life Histories.* New Brunswick, NJ: Rutgers University Press.

MARGARET LOCK

2   Situated Ethics, Culture, and the Brain Death "Problem" in Japan

Science must no longer give the impression it represents a faithful reflection of reality. What it is, rather, is a cultural system . . . specific to a definite time and place.

Wolf Lepenies (1989:64)

ANTHROPOLOGISTS ARE trained to be inherently skeptical of generalizations—to be alert to boundaries, margins, and differences. Most, but not all, of us are "splitters" in Tambiah's idiom (1990); that is, we seek to relativize information by situating it in context. Moreover, to the majority of anthropologists, contextualization intuitively means the situation of knowledge in "cultural" context. But for many thoughtful anthropologists today, the problem of contextualization cannot be dealt with unless two issues are confronted head-on: (1) What do we *mean* by culture, and does this continue to be a useful category? (Similar questions arise with respect to history.) (2) Do we need to examine *all* knowledge and practices, including those that go under the rubric of science, in context; that is, must we subject the truth claims of science and their associated ethical commentaries to epistemological scrutiny? Specific, located practices, not theoretical abstractions, should provide the starting point for such examinations. The focus then becomes one of establishing how competing knowledge claims are legitimized and function in practice and, very importantly, determining what impact they have on the lives of the people they affect most directly. Anthropologists, in contrast perhaps to many philosophers and bioethicists, are wary of taking moral positions. Until recently, the object of their research endeavor has been descriptive rather than prescriptive. Over the past decade, however, certain anthropologists have moved to a position quite close to that of "contextualist morality," as outlined by Hoffmaster (1990), in which morality becomes intelligible "only when the background that makes it possible is considered" (Hoffmaster 1990:250).

39

Contemporary anthropology, certain branches of which are influenced by both hermeneutics and semiotics, is a discipline in which self-reflection about the production of knowledge has become integral to its practice. In particular, the ways in which the knowledge and assumptions of the researcher are inextricably part of the final research product are recognized now. Contextualization is not, therefore, simply an exercise in situating knowledge and practices in a specific locality—in historical and cultural context—rather, it is recognized as an active creation to which the understandings of *both* observer and observed contribute.

Among those who keep abreast of topics in bioethics, most will be familiar with the current situation in Japan, where transplanting solid organs obtained from donors diagnosed as brain dead was prohibited until 1997. Brain death, although a medical diagnosis, was recognized as the end of life in Japan in that year, but only under very specific circumstances. Since 1997 there have been just eight organ procurements from brain dead donors. I have been doing ethnographic research on this topic for approximately twelve years; that is, I have worked to generate a contextualized understanding of the Japanese situation and to translate this understanding into articles written for English language audiences. When I first undertook this research, my more than twenty years of experience in Japan as an anthropologist led me to assume that Japanese culture would in effect account for what is called the "brain death problem" (*nôshi no mondai*) and, further, that such a contextualized explanation could perhaps stimulate some self-reflection on the part of other societies involved with transplant technology about how their respective cultures are implicated (Lock and Honde 1990).

In this chapter, using case studies about the concept of brain death for illustrative purposes, I will attempt to move to a more nuanced approach than the one I took earlier (Lock 1997a, 1997b), an approach in which certain basic concepts, including those of "culture," "society," "nature," "the body," and "technology" are critically examined. Such an exercise provides a cautionary tale about contextualization and suggests, at the minimum, that it is dangerous to argue that essentialized differences—for example, culturally constructed attitudes toward technology and its application—can pass as situated knowledge. In conclusion I will argue for a politicized situational ethics (following Haraway 1991), in which local knowledge is understood as part of history and culture and in which the agency of the people being researched is not only acknowledged, particularly with respect to relationships of power, but also is used to incite a semiotic, reflexive critique of that which is assumed to be natural, normal, and without culture or history—in this particular instance, the relatively easy institutionalization of organ procurement in the United States, Canada, and most European countries.[1]

"Culture" and the Global Economy

The *Guardian Weekly* of 4 August 1996 reprinted an article from the *Washington Post* entitled, "Japanese Are Dying for a Transplant." The article describes the case of twenty-three-year-old Hirofumi Kiuchi, who would have died had he not been flown to Los Angeles for a heart transplant. More than 10,000 Japanese, "many of whom had heart ailments," contributed $380,000 (*Guardian Weekly* 1996). The article is unabashedly partisan in its stance and asserts, among other things, that the situation in Japan has become a national embarrassment. Perhaps it is not surprising that an American journalist writing from Tokyo should summarize the problem as follows: "Citing tradition, culture and religious concerns, Japan has rejected medical advances that have given thousands of critically ill people around the world a second chance at life" (*Guardian Weekly* 1996). What is surprising is the statement Mr. Kiuchi is reported to have made: "I feel that I was supposed to be killed by Japan, by the Japanese government, Japanese tradition, Japanese culture. If I had stayed there I would have died." It seems as though not only the journalist but also the patient is casting the problem as one of "technology versus tradition." What the journalist does not recognize is that although Japanese patients have not been able to undergo transplants using organs from brain dead donors in their own country until very recently, in contrast to recipients living in many other technologically sophisticated societies, it is only in the past four or five years that recipients and potential recipients have become openly vocal in complaining about the situation in Japan. To cast Japanese culture in such a negative light, as does Mr. Kiuchi, has been unusual, although recently the situation has changed.

It is tempting to start from the assumption that a wealthy society with the technological know-how would inevitably foster transplant technology and to dismiss the Japanese situation as an anachronism—as the result of the stubborn weight of "tradition." But can we rely on this journalist in Tokyo? Has she examined her own assumptions about this particular technology? What exactly does she mean by Japanese "culture" and "tradition"? Does she understand that the "brain death problem" has been the most contentious bioethical debate in Japan for three decades, and that more than one thousand monographs and journal and magazine articles have been written on the subject in Japanese? And can we generalize from the words of one citizen, however much his physical condition moves our sympathies? Should we perhaps pay attention to the argument of the Japanese sociologist, Jiro Nudeshima (1991), when he concludes that Japanese "culture" is not at work, but that a lack of trust in doctors is the major reason why brain death went unrecognized for so long as the end of life? But then we must surely ask why Nudeshima does not consider Japanese attitudes toward the medical profession as part of culture? Clearly "culture" and "tradition" serve as interchangeable rhetorical devices and are used to signal the idea that culture works in opposition to the logic of modernity—to the hegemony of science and technology and their associated institutions.

The concept of culture is troubling, particularly for anthropologists who have over the course of this century appropriated it as their key disciplinary category. Recently use of the concept of culture has proliferated across several disciplines—most notably in cultural studies and literary criticism. It has also been invoked liberally in the politics of multiculturalism, a movement that has emerged across North America during the past decade. Many practicing anthropologists have been distressed by, and at times frankly aghast at, how the concept they have honed to a workable consensus has now become "up for grabs," often with crude outcomes. Of particular concern is the way in which the concept frequently is taken as "fact," as though culture is a given reality for which no further explanation is necessary.

Without entering into a complex recapitulation of the argument, let me summarize what I take to be the current position of many anthropologists on the subject of culture. There is concern that culture is used as a "totalizing" concept, one that is particularly amenable to appropriation by those with nationalistic interests. Dominquez argues that culture should be thought of as something invoked, not as something that "is" (1992:23). Along this line, a number of anthropologists now argue that the idea of culture is self-consciously put to work by human communities to assert that their members share an inherited tradition from the past; this reinvented history usually is imagined as one that is uncorrupted by either colonial forces or modern influences. Thus, mythohistory is invoked to create an idealized past out of which culture can be turned into an "exclusionary teleology" (Daniel 1991:8). Some of the contributions to the brain death debate in Japan draw on the notion of culture as an idealized past, a past undominated by Western influences.

The concept of culture is not used solely to emphasize the differences among people. Culture is exclusionary also when it is conceptualized in opposition to nature, where nature is understood as another given, as the "natural" order—that which is not created by human endeavor but by a higher power or, alternatively, through the forces of evolution. It is at this margin, where culture is perceived to encroach on the natural world, that a rupture occurs and becomes a site for the emergence of disputative moralizing discourses. The brain dead body is an ambiguous figure that resides in this space between culture and nature, neither alive nor dead.

In seeking to understand the contemporary world, certain anthropologists are concerned about a further difficulty associated with the concept of culture, namely, that today the world is in a permanent state of flux and transition. Borders and boundaries can no longer easily be demarcated. Arjun Appadurai argues that the central problem of today's global interactions is "the tension between cultural homogenization and cultural heterogenization" (1990:5). By homogenization often it is meant "Americanization" or "commoditization," or both, but such arguments usually fail to recognize a second process, that of indigenization, which takes place simultaneously with homogenization, and jointly works to transform ideas, behaviors, and material goods to "fit" their new locality.

How might an observer utilize the concept of culture as it is imagined in Japan and by outsiders observing Japan? Should it be discarded as fiction? Should it be dropped because it unavoidably creates an essentialized argument? Or can it be of help in trying to contextualize and account for events within the country and the managed flow of knowledge in and out of Japan? My position is that culture is a useful analytical category, provided it is understood as ubiquitous and intrinsic to all social arrangements. The concept encompasses local, tacit, largely unquestioned knowledge and practices, but aspects of culture also can be debated, disputed, and put to work for political ends. Culturally informed values are not distributed equally across populations of people and inevitably are implicated in relationships of power and the maintenance of inequalities. Furthermore, social and institutional arrangements, whatever their purpose and location, are culturally informed. To argue that brain death has never been recognized in Japan as human death because of cultural and religious inhibitions is to reduce a complex, challenging issue to the banal. One could insist equally well, given this line of argument, that the reason brain death was recognized so rapidly in North America and most of Europe is entirely because of local cultural and religious beliefs.

USING CULTURE TO THINK TECHNOLOGY

Bunka (culture) is a concept with a history of several hundred years in Japan. However, the way in which it is most widely imagined at present crystallized in the nineteenth century as a result of sustained contact with Europe, during which time Japanese politicians and intellectuals steeped themselves in the full gamut of European thinking, including evolutionary theory. Throughout the late nineteenth century an eager quest to reproduce Western science and technology "was grounded in [a] sense of cultural certitude" (Najita 1989), an awareness that the "core" or the bass note (*koso*) of Japanese culture would remain unaffected. Technology, self-consciously aligned with the "other" of the "West," was placed in opposition to culture in this discourse and was epitomized by the platitudes *wakon yôsai* (Japanese spirit and Western technology) and *tôyô dôtoku, seiyô gijutsu* (Eastern morality, Western technology). This opposition is different from the culture/nature dichotomy usually associated with Euro/America, in which technology is understood as part of culture designed to "master" nature. In Japan, by contrast, it is often argued that being Japanese entails being in harmony with nature. Thus the culture/nature complex of Japan was, in the nineteenth century, and still often is, routinely set off in rhetorical debates from the cold, rational, culture/technological complex of the West.

Early this century and again, particularly after World War II, internal tension erupted over Japan's increasing technological sophistication and internationalization (Najita 1989). Fears about an imminent collapse of the nation's cultural heritage, in particular its "Westernization," became commonplace, and one reaction was a reassertion of cultural essentialism (Harootunian 1989). Perhaps the dominant theme in internal Japanese debate over the past forty years has been the extent to which it is appropriate or possible to continue to cultivate this sense of uniqueness—of "natural" difference from all other peoples. Not surprisingly, it is usually conservatives who vociferously insist that Japan is inherently different from both the West and other Asian countries. Conservative reconstructions of history suggest that the Japanese continue to be, as they have been from mythological times, "naturally" bonded together as a moral, social, and linguistic unit (Kosaku 1992). Today the majority of Japanese take marked exception to the extreme form of this rhetoric, which slips easily into racism and xenophobia, but it is evident that such a powerful discourse, at times explicitly supported by the government (Gluck 1993; Pyle 1987) and inflamed by trade wars, whaling, and international peace-keeping disputes, cannot easily be dismissed in toto (Cummings 1993; Kalland and Moeran 1992).

For many Japanese commentators, the specter of Westernized individualism, utilitarianism, and superrationalism triggers emotional responses that push them toward a rhetoric of difference, even as they buck at its nationalistic and essentialist underpinnings. This is the discursive background against which the brain death debate is taking place. Appellations such as "tradition," "cultural heritage," and "religion" smack of superstition and premodern sentimentality to many people, but the waters are muddied because Japan repeatedly is described by certain internal commentators and outside observers alike as having undergone a unique form of modernization, one which is distinct from Western capitalism.

When the sociologist Nudeshima, the transplant recipient Kiuchi, the American journalist, and others refer to Japanese culture and tradition, what exactly do they imagine? Given the above discussion, it seems unlikely that they each conceptualize the same entity, or that it has similar implications for them. The comments of Tomoko Abe, a pediatrician employed for many years in a Japanese hospital that specializes in neurological disorders, add yet another dimension to this debate. Abe has spent considerable energy during the past decade working against allowing a diagnosis of brain death to signify human death. She is by no means alone in this activity: Citizen groups in opposition to the recognition of brain death, in one of which Dr. Abe is a member, lawyers, members of the Japanese police force, and a good number of physicians have, between them, managed to ensure that the "brain death problem" remains unresolved.

In discussing her objections with me, Tomoko Abe (personal communication, 1997) emphasized that, in her opinion, the concept of brain death was created primarily for the purpose of facilitating organ transplants. She is emphatic that when a dying person is understood as the focus of both a concerned family and a caring medical team, it is difficult to interpret brain death as the demise of an individual. Abe's opinion is derived, she states, from reflection on her own subjective feelings as a pediatrician:

> The point is not whether the patient is conscious or unconscious [this, for Abe, is the crux of the North American argument about brain death], but whether one *intuitively* understands that the patient is dead. Someone whose color is good, who is still warm, bleeds when cut, and urinates and defecates, is not dead as far as I am concerned. Of course I know that cardiac arrest will follow some hours later—but I think even more significant is the transformation of the warm body into something which is cold and hard—only then do the Japanese really accept death.

In common with the majority of other Japanese doctors I have interviewed on this subject, whether they accept that a diagnosis of brain death can be equated with human death, Tomoko Abe insists that the feelings of family members must be put first, and if, as commonly is believed, the majority of Japanese do not recognize brain death as the end of life, then matters should rest at that. The respirator, without which cardiac arrest would quickly ensue, is not turned off until the family accepts that there will be no recovery—usually four or five days after brain death is medically established. But by this time it is too late for most solid organs to be procured in a usable condition.

Abe herself argues that her response is most probably influenced by the Buddhist heritage of which she, as a Japanese, is a part. Other people I have interviewed say that Japanese opposition to brain death is because of animism, Shintoism, Confucianism, tradition, old-fashioned ideas, and superstition. It is perhaps pertinent to juxtapose the opinion of an American transplant surgeon with that of Tomoko Abe. This surgeon finds that after years of clinical practice, he can no longer dissect organs out of brain dead bodies, but he is unable to verbalize why this is so. To this could be added the words of a Canadian transplant surgeon who declared to me, somewhat sheepishly, that he would be very ill at ease if he should need a heart transplant and find that the organ had been taken out of a criminal. An eminent London lawyer, familiar with the dilemmas posed by a range of biomedical technologies, expressed a similar sentiment when he informed me that the whole business of organ transplants made him "feel queasy" and he would never donate or receive organs. Are these men irrational? Is Tomoko Abe irrational? Are they perhaps *selectively* irrational over certain issues and not others? Or are they simply being human, jibing at the normalization of extraordinary procedures?

One thing is evident. Abe's position cannot be explained away as because of culture or religion, leaving the situation in North America where transplantation has been routinized as the default position—the rational, modern position. As one Japanese informant was quick to point out, the very idea that the donor "lives on" in the recipient clearly is animistic, and although few clinicians accept this metaphor at face value (although it seems many donors and perhaps recipients do [Sharp 1995]), it nevertheless remains a key trope in promoting organ donation in North America and Europe.

Contextualization includes an examination not only of the sites where action takes place, but also of the silences; anything less means that tacit knowledge embedded in dominant discourses remains naturalized. In North America it is appropriate to ask why there was no initial public outcry over the new death located in the brain, created for us by a small group of physicians constituted at Harvard as an ad hoc committee in 1969 (Giacomini 1997). In Japan the pressing question becomes why the voices of those in need of a transplant have not been heard until recently. With this cautionary preamble about the dangers of a facile contextualization and an unproblematized use of the concept of culture, I will turn for the remainder of the chapter to the specifics of the debate about brain death in Japan.

MEDICAL EXPERIMENTATION UNDER FIRE

Shortly after the world's first heart transplant was conducted in South Africa, several attempts were made to carry out the same procedure in other locations. In 1968, just one year after the Barnard case, the thirtieth attempt was made in Sapporo, Hokkaido. As in other locations, the Sapporo procedure initially produced an accolade from the media and was heralded as a dramatic medical triumph. Several months later, however, the physician in charge, Dr. Wada, was arraigned on a murder charge and acquitted only after several years of wrangling. The majority of Japanese believe in retrospect that the patient whose heart was removed was not brain dead, and that the recipient, who died two-and-a-half months after the operation, was not sufficiently in need of a new heart to have undergone the procedure in the first place. As part of the ongoing national debate about brain death, discussion of the case formally was reopened in 1991, and the chairman of the Japanese Medical Association (JMA), testifying before a government committee, reported that twenty-three years before, right after the removal of the supposedly ineffective heart from the recipient patient, it had been tampered with, indicating that the involved doctors apparently had tried to exaggerate the degree of its deterioration. The case is now considered a barbarous piece of medical experimentation carried out by a doctor who received a good portion of his training in America, who now resides in Japan's "untamed hinterland" of Hokkaido, and who is, furthermore, described as self-aggrandizing, that is, not typically Japanese (*Mainichi Shinbun*, "Cover-Up Suspected in First Heart Transplant," 31 March 1991).

In several other organ transplant cases, the Japanese medical profession has not appeared in a good light. Together with the Wada case, they are extensively discussed and criticized in the media and have become iconic for the entire debate. One, for example, involved a highly controversial kidney/pancreas transplant in which organs were removed from a forty-one-year-old woman diagnosed as brain dead and described as mentally incompetent. She earlier had intimated that she wished to donate her heart but no other organs, and her husband had not given permission for her to be a donor (*Mainichi Daily News*, "Organs Removed from Woman without Consent," 24 December 1984).

In 1993, twenty-five years after the first and only liver transplant using a brain dead donor was conducted in Japan, a second effort was made at an emergency medical center outside Osaka. The donor, whose wishes about donation were not known, was declared brain dead. His mother was asked whether donation would be acceptable and, under what was reported as considerable pressure, she consented. The case rapidly was leaked to the media, and the involved medical team publicly was chided for its "aggressive" behavior. The media reported that the physicians unhooked the respirator, waited one minute following cardiac arrest before starting to perfuse the liver, removed it, and then transported it to Kyûshû, 400 miles away, where it was transplanted into a patient who was not immunologically compatible with the donor.

The wife of the recipient, at her own insistence, appeared on television to thank the donor and the transplant team. The nonfiction writer Michi Nakajima, also trained in law and well known for her antipathy to accepting brain death as human death, has asserted that this case is as bad as the notorious "Wada" episode. She claims that the donor *proba-bly* had a beating heart when the liver was removed, and that the involved physicians simply said the heart had stopped beating to pla-cate the authorities and the public. Moreover, insists Nakajima (1994), the donor's mother was in a state of shock after the event and did not fully understand that donation was being requested. Furthermore, the physicians did not first establish whether death was accidental, in which case the police should have been called in for an autopsy report before any organs were removed. The University of Tokyo Patients' Rights Group, in which Tomoko Abe participates, called for a public inquiry into this case. In all, twenty physicians in Japan have been charged with murder in connection with organ procurement. In 1998, eight unsettled cases were finally thrown out of court, but shortly there-after one new charge of murder was made against a doctor in Okinawa (*Asahi Shinbun*, "Izoku to ishi tsutawaranu kokoro" [The Deceased's Family and Doctor Failed to Communicate], 24 March 1998).

These cases indicate the tenacity and determination of opposition groups. That such cases constantly are given extensive media attention means that the Japanese public, including medical professionals, cannot avoid questioning what goes on behind the closed doors of operating theaters and in intensive care units. There is plenty of skepticism about the accuracy of media reporting in Japan, but the barrage of television programs, newspaper reports, and magazine articles cannot be set aside without some disquiet. Some mix of culture, politics, corruption, and professional hubris seems to be driving these incidents. No matter what incites them, these case studies provide enormous incentive for public debate about the treatment of brain dead patients. Without such inci-dents the Japanese public would be in the same position as the North American public—for the most part uninformed and uninterested.

I have been told by one pediatric intensivist working in the American Midwest that he has had to throw transplant surgeons out of his unit when they come "trolling" for organs. One does not have to go far to find other disquieting stories in North America. The implementation a few years ago of the Pittsburgh protocol to procure organs from non-heart-beating cadaver donors, subsequently adopted in other institutions, certainly is cause for concern (Arnold and Youngner 1993). My hunch is that if the media in North America were as intrusive and aggressive on this subject as the Japanese media are, organ donation rates might well decline here. Perhaps we should ask what it is about our "culture" that makes us—the media, the public, health care professionals—turn away from possible abuses of patients with severe brain trauma.

CONTESTED DEFINITIONS OF DEATH

A law permitting corneal transplantation in Japan was enacted in 1958. The first definition of brain death was formulated by the Japan Electroencephaly Association in 1974. Probably in response to the much publicized case of the mentally impaired patient cited above, the Life Ethics Problem Study Parlimentarians League, composed of twenty-eight Diet members and forty-five other professionals, was established in 1985, and after one year this group endorsed the need for legislation about brain death (Feldman 1996). In the same year, the Ministry of Health and Welfare set up a Brain Death Advisory Council, the final report of which contains the definition of brain death used in Japan today (Kôseishô 1985). This report is explicit, however, that "death cannot be judged by brain death." Nevertheless, the diagnosis frequently is made, and although it is not usually a signal to turn off the respirator, it serves to prepare relatives for an impending death (Ohi et al. 1986). Relatives usually are informed that the patient is "almost brain dead" (*hobo nôshi no jotai*) or in a "hopeless" condition, even when attending physicians are convinced that the patient is brain dead.

The Ministry's report spurred other groups to make pronouncements about their positions. In January 1988, after two years of meetings by a working group, the directors of the JMA voted unanimously to accept brain death as the end of human life, but despite this decision, a lack of agreement remains among representatives of the various medical specialties and also among individual physicians, who are deeply divided on the issue. The politically outspoken Japan Association of Psychiatrists and Neurologists (some of whose 6,900 members are responsible for making brain death diagnoses) fears, for example, that equating brain death with human death will lead to a slippery slope on which the handicapped, mentally impaired, and disadvantaged will be at risk of being prematurely diagnosed in a greedy desire to get their organs. In their 1988 report this group emphasized the difficulty of precisely determining when brain function is irreversibly lost. The society for specialists in emergency medicine, also directly involved in diagnosing brain death, took until 1994 to reach an agreement that brain death is equivalent to human death (*Nihon Kyûkyû Igakukai rinji kai* 1994).

As a result of the unresolved debate, copiously documented by the media, the government felt compelled in late 1989 to set up a Special Cabinet Committee on Brain Death and Organ Transplants to bring about closure. This committee, composed of fifteen members from various walks of life, was charged to make a report to the Prime Minister by 1991, and its formation signaled to the public that the government was ready to support a move to legalize brain death as the end of life. The group was divided so deeply that for a while it appeared it would never produce anything more than an interim report, but in January 1992 a final report was made public. In principle the members should have reached a consensus, but they could not achieve it. The majority position was that brain death is equivalent to human biological death and that it can be diagnosed accurately using what is known as the Takeuchi Standard (virtually the same criteria used in North America), which had already been adopted by the Ministry of Health and Welfare. The majority report asserted that it is "rational" to consider brain death as the end of life, and therefore sensible to accept it as equivalent to social and legal death.

The committee members who wrote the minority report wish to have what they describe as the "social and cultural" aspects of the brain death problem fully debated; in their opinion the discussion had been largely confined to "scientific" information, which they believe to be inadequate (*Yomiuri Shinbun*, "Nôshi ishoku yonin o saigo tôshin" [Final Report Approves of Brain Death, Organ Transplants], 23 January 1992). The public was kept fully apprised of who appeared before the committee, and many of those who testified, including certain scientists and doctors, argued against the acceptance of brain death; nevertheless, the majority of the committee eventually supported its recognition.

In the meantime the Japan Federation of Bar Associations (*Nichibenren*) has maintained its position of the past twenty-five years against accepting brain death as equivalent to human death (in contrast to the stance of equivalent legal associations in North America). This organization repeatedly has expressed concern for the "sanctity of life" and about possible "medical experimentation." The federation also has pointed out that there may be unforeseen consequences in connection with inheritance claims, and they noted that a lack of public consensus on the issue is a major stumbling block (*Asahi Shinbun,* "'Nôshi wa shi to mitomeru.' Nichibenren ikensho rincho o hihan jinken shingai no osore" ["'Recognition of Brain Death as Death.' Fear of Violation of Human Rights in the Opinion of the Japanese Confederation of Lawyers"], 21 September 1992). The day following the announcement of the Cabinet Committee report, the Ministry of Justice, the National Police Agency, and the Public Prosecutor's Office all reiterated their continued resistance to recognizing brain death as the end of individual life.

The Patients' Rights Committee, lawyers, the police, several television program producers, and many authors of newspaper articles and books on the subject of brain death, together with many medical professionals, appear to be publicly contesting the authority of transplant surgeons, for they believe that in the rush to retrieve organs, the process of dying will be curtailed or death will even be misdiagnosed. Those organizations and individuals who form the opposition in the debate about the brain death problem explicitly object to the secrecy and arrogance of certain members of the Japanese medical profession and point out that patients and their families are vulnerable to exploitation when left in their hands:

Many of these opponents are at the same time pushing for informed consent, which is far from routine in Japan (Leflar 1996), together with candid disclosures of diagnoses and prognoses to patients and frank discussions of their conditions. Although at one level this contest is a debate about the accuracy and consistency of medical decision making, it is also a challenge to the hegemony of invested authority, authority exerted in what several of the challengers characterize as a traditional Japanese way, whereby subjects are rendered passive and expected to comply with medical regimens without question.

Members of opposition groups are by no means always opposed to organ transplants (although a good number are), but they genuinely are concerned about paternalism, professional self-interest, that informed consent is not thoroughly institutionalized, a lack of equity in the distribution of organs, and corruption. Although Japan has had a socialized health care system for more than half a century, surgeons (and other specialists) are nevertheless accustomed to receiving substantial gifts for services rendered. Members of the public often read about cases of bribery in the medical profession. Many people when talking to me have said quite simply that the transplant enterprise is "not fair."

The opposition to brain death also is driven in part by false information, much of it about what is purported to have happened in North America. For example, what I assume are blatantly inaccurate reports have been made about America, where, it is contended, poor Black families sell the bodies of their deceased children to doctors so that their organs can be harvested (Amano 1987). Japanese citizens also view programs and read extensively about the sale of organs in other parts of Asia, countries to which Japanese patients in need of transplants go in desperation. The brain death problem is debated against this background buzz of information and misinformation.

Those in Japan who wish to break the impasse in the brain death debate often dismiss members of the opposition as prisoners of the past, enthralled by the culture of tradition. This is clearly not the case in general, although among those who are opposed some draw on the notions of culture, tradition, or religion to justify their arguments, and a few are indeed reactionary. The majority of the opposition, however, are concerned primarily with general issues of justice and have intentionally used the issues around brain death to make their case.

REACHING PUBLIC CONSENSUS

Taking place in concert with government, professional, and media discussions is the most persistent search for a national consensus (*kokuminteki gôi*) among the Japanese public that has occurred to date on any subject. Between 1983 and 1996 there have been at least fourteen national surveys and numerous smaller ones about brain death and organ transplants. Over the years the number of people who have come to recognize brain death as the end of life has increased from 29 percent to almost 50 percent. In all the surveys a paradox is evident, however, in that although many people approve of organ retrieval from brain dead patients, they do not accept brain death as the end of life. It seems that the Japanese public is willing to allow transplants to take place, even though many think they would not personally be comfortable with participating in these procedures (*Asahi Shinbun*, "Nôshi shi toshite 53%" [Brain Death as Death 53%], 1 October 1996).

Opponents of brain death usually draw on the results of opinion polls because frequently it is reiterated that public consensus must be reached before brain death can be nationally recognized. Nevertheless, one is left with the feeling, voiced by many members of the Japanese public, that the whole exercise of repeatedly surveying the nation is a farce, and that the idea of trying to achieve a simple consensus on such an inflammatory subject is meaningless.

In the autumn of 1994, a private member's bill was submitted to the Diet calling for brain death to be established as the end of life and for the removal of organs from brain dead patients, with the consent of family members, to be legalized. The bill did not require that the patients' wishes be known, only that they should be "surmised" (*sontaku suru*) by close relatives. The bill was not discussed before parliament was dissolved. Those who are adamantly opposed to redefining death were quick to criticize the bill. Active opposition came from the Japanese Association for Philosophical and Ethical Research in Medicine, which believes that the human rights of brain dead persons inevitably will be violated. Other critics argued that grieving family members are vulnerable, and that if the will of the patient is not known, there should be no option of either turning off the respirator or asking for organ donation. Other critics insisted that neither the law, nor public officials, nor the medical profession should have the last word about the recognition of death, because the opinion of every citizen is equally valid on such a matter.

The previous government's Minister of Health and Welfare announced in 1994 that his ministry would not oppose using brain dead donors' organs for transplantation, even before a bill made its way through the Diet. Not surprisingly, the Japan Society for Transplantation concurred with this position, but the actions of a team of doctors at Yokohama General Hospital produced a strong current of criticism among dissenters, both within the JMA and among the Japanese public. This team of surgeons reported that early in 1994 kidneys had been removed from four brain dead patients before their hearts had stopped beating and were then transplanted into eight waiting recipients. Yokohama General Hospital is a large, urban, tertiary care center, but it has no ethics committee and does not meet the requirements set out by the Health and Welfare Ministry for an organ transplant center. Critics have pointed out that only the transplant surgeons were involved in the decision making and in obtaining family consent. After this incident a heated debate occurred in the media about whether the controversial clause in the failed bill allowing family members to surmise patients' wishes could ever be acted on appropriately should such a bill be passed.

In June 1994, the mother of a young nurse whose kidney had been removed following her death filed suit with the Osaka Bar Association claiming that doctors cared more about the kidney than they did about saving her daughter's life. Doctors had not informed the woman that her daughter was brain dead and instead stressed that the kidney was needed for another patient. Cases such as this suggest that major gaps in expectations about care and in communication between doctors and patients' families continue in Japan. Many informants spontaneously have commented to me that "we are not yet ready for brain death in Japan."

PUBLIC COMMENTARY ON THE BRAIN DEATH PROBLEM

Numerous Japanese television programs, magazine articles, and best-selling books repeatedly have cast doubt on whether death can be understood as a clearly diagnosable event (see, for example, Hirosawa 1992; Komatsu 1993). It also has been argued in books and the media that irreversibility is difficult to establish conclusively, and cases have been noted outside of Japan where mistakes evidently have been made. As well, some commentators question whether a lack of integrated brain function does indeed indicate death.

One highly influential journalist, Takashi Tachibana (1991), author of several books and coordinator of television programs on the subject of brain death and organ transplants, emphasizes that brain cells continue to live even when the brain as a whole has no integrated function. Mr. Tachibana dwells in all his media presentations on the "liveliness" of a brain dead individual. A Saturday evening prime time program, aired in 1990 and hosted by him, started out, for example, with shots of a beautiful, active, six-year-old child who was born, viewers were informed, from a brain dead mother. "How *can* a brain dead body not be living," asked Mr. Tachibana rhetorically? He and other writers, together with the majority of more than fifty Japanese citizens I have interviewed on the subject, including health care professionals and the public, inevitably point out that blood flows when the bodies of the brain dead are cut, their hair and nails grow, their basic metabolism continues, and live birth is possible from a brain dead woman. The majority also emphasize that the brain dead remain warm and appear as though they were sleeping; they point out that nursing care and expressions of love and concern by the family of the dying involve touching, holding hands, and massaging. There is agreement that it goes against "basic human feelings" to assume that a warm body is dead, and many assert that the average Japanese family could not in good conscience abandon a dying relative to a transplant team.

As Tomoko Abe, the pediatrician, made clear, the *presence* of death is not denied in arguments such as these, but what is being explicitly suggested is that the *process* of dying is transformed arbitrarily into a technologically determined time, as early as possible along the spectrum of biological demise. There is concern that family members cannot adjust easily to a medically determined diagnosis of irreversible brain function, and that they are likely to assume that death is being declared before the process has been completed.

Other writers, taking a slightly different tack, stress that because brain death can be determined only by trained medical personnel— because it is *mienai shi* (death that cannot be seen)—it represents a radical departure from the usual situation where the family participates fully in the dawning recognition of the process. Making integrated brain function the measure of death ensures that the family is pushed to the sidelines, rendered passive, and left entirely at the mercy of medical decision making (Nakajima 1985).

Masahiro Morioka (1991), a philosopher and bioethicist, has argued (drawing on Bentham's panopticon) that the intensive care unit is in some ways similar to a modern prison, in that patients are monitored from a central nursing station and are for the most part separated from family members. He suggests that brain death should be analyzed as more than a medical decision about the condition of the brain, and that the patient is best understood as existing at the loci of human relationships. This social unit should be the starting point for determining the acceptance or otherwise of brain death as the end of life.

Kunio Yanagida is the son of Japan's most celebrated cultural historian of the same name, who died some years ago. Recently, the younger Yanagida galvanized the Japanese public by publishing two widely circulated articles followed by a book about his own son, who tried to commit suicide and was taken to hospital where he was diagnosed as brain dead (Yanagida 1994, 1995, 1996). Yanagida reports that his family experienced nothing but sympathetic support from the doctor in charge of the case.

Yanagida had found his son, Yojiro, in his bedroom with an electrical cord wound around his neck. Yojiro was rushed to hospital, but his condition worsened over the next three days, and eventually he was diagnosed as brain dead. Yanagida recalls that during those first days his eldest son had asked the doctor if he could wipe away his brother's tears because "he seemed to be crying a lot." The doctor was sympathetic but explained that this was purely a physical phenomenon, not an expression of emotion. "We don't know why this happens," he replied. Yanagida writes that he started to think about organ donation while seated at the bedside because together with his son he had watched a television program on the subject, and his son had at the time expressed an interest in helping other people. Yanagida recalls that as he held his son's hand and whispered his name, his son's face was "bright and warm," and he "couldn't bear the idea" of someone putting a knife into his son's body and taking out the heart.

Yanagida reports that he became confused as to what brain death really signifies: Was his son indeed a corpse, or was he still suspended between life and death? Four days after the brain death diagnosis, upon reading his son's diaries in which he expressed sadness at being of no use to anyone, Yanagida came to an understanding that it was his duty to "complete" his son's life. On the fifth day all treatment was stopped. When, several days later, his heart stopped beating, Yojiro's kidneys were removed for transplant. These published reflections poignantly reveal the emotional struggle of someone precipitated into grief over sudden death. But they also express a thoughtful awareness of the dilemma the Japanese medical profession experiences with this particular technology, and they reveal a sensitivity to those waiting for organs. Nevertheless, there can be little doubt that these articles and the book consolidated the majority opinion in Japan that families should not be rushed into accepting death the moment various tests reveal that a patient is brain dead.

The Japanese media and various magazine articles have raised doubts also about misdiagnosis by arguing that brain death and persistent vegetative state (PVS) cannot be distinguished easily (almost no clinicians in Japan or elsewhere agree with such claims), followed by examples of patients who make partial, and occasionally complete, recoveries from PVS. Three or four hospitals in Japan specialize in the treatment of PVS patients, and one such hospital where intensive nursing care is employed as the prime treatment modality has been the subject of a moving national television program. This type of coverage, when coupled with media reporting that emphasizes medical errors, means that promoters of organ transplants have to battle constantly against the tide of media manipulated popular opinion, reinforced by the opinions of a number of very influential *hyôronka* (intellectuals who appear in the media specially to critique contemporary issues).

DISCOURSE ON SOCIAL DEATH

In Japan, as we have seen, biological death usually is understood as a process, not a point in time, a view with which individuals living in societies where death remains familiar would no doubt agree. Moreover, many Japanese commentators distinguish between biological and social death—the latter is believed to take place some time after the demise of the physical body. Interviews I conducted with fifty urban Japanese men and women made it clear that concern about the fate of the body after biological death may well contribute to a reluctance on the part of some people both to donate and to receive organs. Everyone with whom I talked stated that they no longer participate in the elaborate prewar ancestor system with its complex set of formal rituals involving the extended family over many years. Nevertheless, over half of the respondents indicated that they carry out regular, often daily, rituals in their homes and at the graves of deceased parents and grandparents. Most pointed out that family and societal obligations require that the bodies and memory of deceased family members be treated with respect.

A 1981 survey showed that between 60 percent and 70 percent of Japanese believe that when and where one is born and dies are determined by destiny, something that should not be changed by human intervention (Maruyama, Fumi, and Hasashi 1981). In a recent survey, 40 percent responded that they believe in the continued existence after death of *reikon* (soul/spirit) (Woss 1992). This same survey showed that among young people aged sixteen to twenty-nine, belief in the survival of the soul is particularly prevalent, and it is well documented that Japanese of all ages are now undergoing a revival of interest in animism.

From an analysis of the very moving narratives provided by relatives of victims of the Japan Air Lines crash in the mountains of Gunma prefecture in 1985, the anthropologist Namihira concluded that the spirit of the deceased often is anthropomorphized and is believed to experience the same feelings as do the living. Hence relatives have an obligation to make the spirit happy and comfortable. The relatives agreed that it is important for a dead body to be brought home and that a corpse should be complete (*gotai manzoku*); otherwise the spirit will suffer and may cause harm to the living. Namihira cites the results of a 1983 questionnaire administered by a committee set up to encourage the donation of bodies for medical research: Out of 690 respondents, 66 percent stated that cutting into dead bodies is repulsive, or cruel, or both and shows a lack of respect for the dead (Namihira 1988). Against these figures, the number of people agreeing to autopsies has increased steadily in recent years, as well as the number of people willing to go abroad to obtain organ transplants, and there has been an increasing recognition among the public of brain death as the end of life. Clearly the population's attitudes toward the dying and the recently dead remain deeply divided, and many people would, in any case, probably state one position in response to a survey and act differently when personally confronted with suffering.

It is noteworthy that in Oregon certain families refused to cooperate with autopsies because they believed the "patient" had already suffered enough (Perkins and Tolle 1992), and an age-stratified Swedish study among 1,950 individuals obtained similar results (Sanner 1994). After air disasters, family members, regardless of their culture of origin, exhibit deep concern that every effort should be made to recover the bodies of victims. It should perhaps also be recalled that a recent study in the United States showed that more than 50 percent of those surveyed believe in angels. These responses suggest that there is no deep cultural divide among human groups when coping with death and the afterlife, especially when death is not anticipated. In North America, however, no culturally elaborated vocabulary is in common use to buffer these concerns, suggesting that although they may be widespread, they are likely to remain inchoate.

In contrast, in Japan the boundary between the social and the natural worlds has never been defined rigidly—ancestors were and often continue to be immortalized as entities who act on the everyday world.

Through ritual enactments ancestors eventually become part of an animized natural order, forming a vital bridge between the spiritual, social, and natural domains. This approach to death is grist for the mill of commentators (both inside and outside Japan) who wish to signal that "tradition" and the "old moral order," replete with their conservative patriarchal outlook, are intact and functioning in the Japan of late modernity. Many of the exchanges characteristic of the emotionally charged brain death debate implicitly turn around this point, for to argue against redefining death lands one squarely within this conservative stronghold unless the argument is couched exceedingly carefully. In fact, though, many of those in opposition groups, as noted above, are concerned with the basic rights of individuals and with questions of justice—moral issues central to a modern outlook on the world. Moderate opponents find themselves squeezed, therefore, between those who argue that any rational, scientific mind would accept a redefinition of death, and extreme opponents who usually invoke nationalistic reasons for their recalcitrance. Many of these extremists argue in effect that brain death is "unnatural" and therefore not appropriate for Japan.

There is another major facet to this dispute that it is not possible to develop in this chapter; namely, that it is not simply attitudes toward the dying and dead that are operative in Japan, but also attitudes connected to gift giving. Living related organ donation is not a cause for public concern, but certain commentators question the appropriateness of altruistic donation of organs by strangers. Japan has a remarkably refined system of gift giving, one that is in essence an obligatory system of ongoing exchange of goods and services. Entering into any kind of formalized relationship with people beyond the family involves the giving and receiving of gifts of specified value on regular occasions. This system continues to be used widely in the Japanese economy, in the various institutions where professional services are available, and among families and communities. The result is that the "tyranny of the gift" (Fox and Swazey 1992) is everpresent in Japanese society. The idea of receiving a gift as precious as a human organ is overwhelming to contemplate for most people, because the reciprocal obligations incurred by the family of the recipient would be too hard to bear. Although anonymity in theory provides protection against actually having to fulfill such obligations, it does not relieve a recipient family of enormous feelings of guilt.

This value system imposes an additional burden on those who wish to break the impasse created by the brain death problem. Not only does it make patients hesitant about becoming a transplant recipient, it also raises darker concerns, for, as noted above, doctors routinely receive gifts, monetary and otherwise, in advance of services rendered. Many commentators fear that organs may be donated to individual doctors as gifts or, alternatively, that money may be paid to a surgeon to become a favored potential organ recipient.

INDIVIDUAL SUFFERING AND THE POLITICS OF MORALITY

The present dilemma for progressive-minded thinkers in Japan debating the ethics of the brain death problem is how to dispose of the remnants of patriarchy and patronage—the reactionary parts of the Confucian heritage—without drawing on a language that single-mindedly further entrenches the Western values of individual autonomy and rights. As one pediatrician recently put it: "Why should we mindlessly imitate Westerners? We would only be turning ourselves into white Westerners with Asian faces" (*Newsweek Nihon Han* 1993). Not surprisingly, to regular observers of Japan the debate is overwhelmingly secular, one in which representatives of the dominant religious organizations are absent, with the sole exception of the aggressive Buddhist sect of Sokka Gakkai (Becker 1993).

Although the fate of the individuals whose lives are directly involved arouses genuine passion, remarkably little has been heard until recently from patients and their families, whether they be potential donors or recipients. However, a woman whose daughter will soon require a liver transplant, when interviewed by *Newsweek* for its Japanese edition, complained, "Why do we have to suffer just because we have the misfortune to be Japanese?" (*Newsweek Nihon Han* 1993). Only since the beginning of 1994, the year in which an international conference on organ transplantation was deliberately staged in Japan by surgeons keen to demonstrate the worth of their knowledge and skills, has the fate of those patients not able to receive transplants, together with those who have gone abroad to obtain organs, started to capture the imaginations of the media and the Japanese public.

Thus far, though, the brain death problem has not been primarily about individual human suffering. Rather it is a manifestation of the struggle by citizens and activists from a range of political persuasions over moral order in contemporary Japan, which inevitably involves a discussion, often implicit, about the relationship of nature to culture. Those who recognize brain death as the end of life usually accept a modernist ideology of technologically driven progress in the relief of human suffering, whereas some of those against the brain death diagnosis embrace an argument about the essential difference of Japan and exhibit concerns about a perceived loss of moral order. The majority, however, lie in the soft center, where they seek to support a tempered use of technology, one in which individuals are not subject to exploitation. Because many activists believe that Japan remains a feudal society with respect to power relations, they have spoken out against accepting brain death as the end of life and have ignored the pleas of those who might benefit from transplant technology. Slowly and painfully a middle ground that gives more prominence to accounts of individual suffering is emerging. Even when the suffering of potential organ recipients is recognized, however, activists do not necessarily agree that transplants are an unequivocal good: The Buddhist admonition not to crave that which belongs to others is often cited by opponents (in contrast, advocates sometimes note that Buddhism encourages individuals to sacrifice themselves for others in need). Above all, it is extremists on both sides of the argument, but particularly those in opposition, who remain most influential, for it is they who thus far have captured the imagination of the media.

In April 1997, after thirty years of vituperative public debate, two bills were presented once again to the lower house of the Diet, one of which eventually passed with a sizeable majority. Amid a whirlwind of opposition activities, the upper house of the Diet passed a modified version of the bill, and it became law in October 1997. The bill states that organs may be retrieved from a brain dead patient provided that the patient (at least fifteen years of age) has previously given written consent, and that the family does not overrule the declared wish. If no advance directive exists or if the family is opposed to donation, a brain dead patient will continue to receive medical care until the family and medical team agree to terminate treatment and turn off the ventilator. In other words, brain death is recognized only for those patients and their families who wish to donate organs. It is not recognized as death in the case of any other patient, even one diagnosed as brain dead. Numerous people in Japan are highly critical of the ambiguity built into this new law (Hirano 1997). And as of the summer of the year 2000, only eight transplants using organs procured from brain dead donors have been performed.

The Japanese hospital system still must undergo a major restructuring before it can participate successfully in a national transplant program. At present hospitals are exceedingly competitive, and there is little or no cooperation among specialists in different hospitals or even across specialties within the same hospital. Simply obtaining two independent opinions about a brain death case currently is difficult in many facilities. It seems it is not only the Japanese public that is not ready for brain death, but also many members of the medical profession, some of whom remain highly critical of the system in which they work and concerned about malpractice on the part of their colleagues.

TOWARD A SITUATED ETHICS

From the outset in documenting the brain death problem in Japan, I have made efforts to situate my analysis and my arguments in cultural context. I have increasingly become hesitant about using culture as an explanatory device, however, because of the essentialist way in which this concept is so often wielded, whether by Japanese citizens or outside observers. More than with any other research I have done in Japan, conversations about brain death have forced me to appreciate how much the West is present at most interviews I conduct, as a ghost hovering over my shoulder, affecting what people say and how they phrase it. When talking to a Japanese audience recently, it became clear to me in the question period that discussion would be more productive if it did not so often take place against the background of a barely disguised dichotomy between a mythologized, homogenized Japan and a mythologized, homogenized West.

There is no doubt in my mind that Japanese tradition—animism, Buddhism, Confucianism, group-oriented social relations, attitudes toward nature, and so on—influences the arguments about death and organ transplants. I would venture to say, though, that rather than tradition, it is concerns about modernity (which is not simply the counterpoint to tradition) that drive most of the objections to brain death in Japan. It is also clear that politics are deeply implicated, both within the medical profession and in society at large. Various facets of tradition are selectively called upon, often to reinforce certain political arguments and at other times to demolish them. Furthermore, many people create scientific arguments, believing that such arguments are entirely rational and culture-free. Some of these arguments are designed to promote the transplant enterprise, others to prohibit it. Many, but not all, of those who create scientific arguments actively reject tradition and oppose it to science. Others ignore tradition and culture entirely, and yet others are sensitive to the fact that values infuse all debates, even those defined as scientific. Certain analysts in this last group have started to create cogent arguments that identify the ways in which values are embedded in the North American transplant enterprise.

Clearly culture explains very little unless its use is contextualized carefully, and the same holds for the concepts of nature, society, technology, and so on; none can be taken as an unexamined given. It is particularly important to extend this insight to those geographical locations, notably North America, that thus far have been exempt from such scrutiny and have remained bastions of rational, technological progress, locations where the word "culture," except when referring to the "high" culture of the arts, is almost never applied except to "ethnic minorities."

A situated ethics demands not only that all forms of debate be contextualized, but also that the researcher be made visible—a God's-eye position cannot be countenanced. Despite deep involvement with this topic for several years, no amount of reflection assists me in taking a stable position. Without doing the work in Japan, I would, no doubt, have continued assuming that organ transplants are an incontrovertible good. I no longer believe this to be the case, but having interviewed many organ recipients, both in Canada and Japan, I know that many lives have been improved and actually lengthened, sometimes for many years, by organ transplants. I also know that many others experience only a brief remission before dying or, in the case of kidney transplants, returning to dialysis. I have concluded that statistical survival rates are not helpful in trying to take a personal position, and that extended conversations with those who have experienced this technology are much more useful. I remain unable to predict, with confidence, how I would react if I needed a transplant, or what my response would be if a family member needed one. This suggests to me that polls that purport to investigate public opinion about emotional, life-threatening issues such as transplants may not be of much value. *Perhaps* the response of an

American physician who had recently watched several people die after liver transplants, and who now states that he will never let any of his family members go through such a procedure, is more insightful.

Similarly, I cannot state whether I would have donated the organs of a child of mine had they become brain dead (and I will never have to face this enormous decision, my children now being adults). I suspect that in the event I would have done so, but I cannot be sure, and I certainly cannot advocate that other people should be strongly encouraged to do so.

To me the most challenging intellectual question no longer concerns the Japanese dispute, where the paradoxes and ambiguities associated with brain death and organ transplants lie exposed. As a result of having considered the Japanese case, the burning question for me has become one of explaining why something so profound as a medically engineered proclamation about a new death produced so few ripples in North America, and why the ethical debate here takes off from a so-called shortage of organs (see Lock: in press).

NOTES

Acknowledgment: The research on which this paper is based is funded by the Social Sciences and Humanities Research Council of Canada (SSHRC).

1. In several European countries, notably Denmark and Sweden, this process was not accomplished with ease.

REFERENCES

Amano, K. 1987. Noshi of kangaeru, zoki ishoku to no kanren no naka de (Thoughts on brain death in connection with organ transplants). *Gekkan Naashingu* 15:1949–1953.

Appadurai, Arjun. 1990. Disjuncture and Difference in the Global Cultural Economy. *Public Culture* 2:1–24.

Arnold, Robert, and Stuart Youngner. 1993. The Dead Donor Rule: Should We Stretch It, Bend It, or Abandon It? *Kennedy Institute of Ethics Journal* 3:263–278.

Becker, Carl. 1993. *Breaking the Circle: Death and the Afterlife in Buddhism.* Carbondale, IL: Southern Illinois University Press.

Cummings, Bruce. 1993. Japan's Position in the World System. In *Postwar Japan as History,* ed. A. Gordon, 34–95. Berkeley: University of California Press.

Daniel, Valentine. 1991. *Is There a Counterpoint to Culture? The Wertheim Lecture 1991.* Amsterdam: Centre for Asian Studies.

Dominquez, Virginia R. 1992. Invoking Culture: The Messy Side of "Cultural Politics." *South Atlantic Quarterly* 91:19–42.

Feldman, Eric A. 1996. Body Politics: The Impasse Over Brain Death and Organ Transplantation in Japan. In *Containing Health Care Costs in Japan*, eds. John Campbell and Naoki Ikegami, 234–247. Ann Arbor: University of Michigan Press.

Fox, Renée, and J. Swazey. 1992. *Spare Parts: Organ Replacement in American Society*. New York: Oxford University Press.

Giacomini, Mita. 1997. A Change of Heart and a Change of Mind? Technology and the Redefinition of Death in 1968. *Social Science and Medicine* 44: 1465–1482.

Gluck, Carol. 1993. The Past in the Present. In *Postwar Japan as History*, ed. A. Gordon, 64- 95. Berkeley: University of California Press.

Haraway, Donna. 1991. Situated Knowledge: The Science Question in Feminism and the Privilege of Partial Perspective. In *Simians, Cyborgs and Women: The Reinvention of Nature*, ed. Donna Haraway, 183–202. New York: Routledge.

Harootunian, H. D. 1989. Visible Discourse/Invisible Ideologies. In *Postmodernism and Japan*, eds. M. Miyoshi and H. D. Harootunian, 63–92. Durham, NC: Duke University Press.

Hirano, Ryuichi. 1997. Sanpo ichiryozon teki kaiketsu: Soft landing no tame no zanteiteki sochi (A solution that makes each party lose an equal amount: Tentative measure for soft landing). *Jurist* 1121:30–38.

Hirosawa, Kôshichirô. 1992. Tachiba kara mita nôshi to shinzô ishoku (Brain death and heart transplants from the point of view of a circulatory system specialist). In *Nôshi to zôki-ishoku* (Brain Death and Organ Transplants), ed. Takeshi Umehara, 62–80. Tokyo: Asahi Shinbunsha.

Hoffmaster, Barry. 1990. Morality and the Social Sciences. In *Social Science Perspectives on Medical Ethics*, ed. George Weisz, 241–260. Dordrecht: Kluwer Academic.

Kalland, Arne, and Brian Moeran. 1992. *Japanese Whaling: End of an Era?* London: Curzon.

Komatsu, Yoshihiko. 1993. Sentaku gijutsu to nôshironsô no shikaku (The blind spot in advanced technology and brain death debates). *Gendai Shisô* 21: 198–212.

Kosaku, Yoshino. 1992. *Cultural Nationalism in Contemporary Japan: A Sociological Inquiry*. London: Routledge.

Kôseishô. 1985. "Kôseishô kenkyûhan ni yoru nôshi no hantei kijun" (Brain death determination criteria of the Ministry of Health and Welfare). Tokyo: Author.

Leflar, Robert B. 1996. Informed Consent and Patients' Rights in Japan. *Houston Law Review* 3:1–112.

Lepenies, Wolf. 1989. The Direction of the Disciplines: The Future of the Universities. *Comparative Criticism* 11:51–70.

Lock, Margaret. 1997a. Displacing Suffering: The Reconstruction of Death in North America and Japan. In *Social Suffering*, eds. Arthur Kleinman, Veena Das, and Margaret Lock, 207–244. Berkeley: University of California Press.

———. 1997b. The Unnatural as Ideology: Contesting Brain Death in Japan. In *Japanese Images of Nature: Cultural Perspectives*, eds. Pamela Asquith and Arne Kalland, 121–144. Cambridge: Cambridge University Press.

————. In press. *Twice Dead: Organ Transplants and the Reinvention of Death*. Berkeley: University of California Press.

Lock, Margaret, and Christine Honde. 1990. Reaching Consensus about Death: Heart Transplants and Cultural Identity in Japan. In *Social Science Perspectives on Medical Ethics*, ed. George Weisz, 99–119. Dordrecht: Kluwer Academic.

Maruyama, Kumiko, Hayashi Fumi, and Kamisasa Hisashi. 1981. A Multivariate Analysis of Japanese Attitudes toward Life and Death. *Behaviormetrika* 10:37–48.

Morioka, Masahiro. 1991. *Nôshi no Hito* (Brain dead people). Tokyo: Fukutake Shoten.

Najita, Tetsuo. 1989. On Culture and Technology in Postmodern Japan. In *Postmodernism and Japan*, eds. M. Miyoshi and H. D. Harootunian, 3–20. Durham, NC: Duke University Press.

Nakajima, Michi. 1985. *Mienai shi: Nôshi to zôki ishoku* (Invisible death: Brain death and organ transplants). Tokyo: Bungei Shunju.

————. 1994. Noshi-Ripô wo isogaseta Kyushû Daigaku igakubu no Kanzô ishoku hôdo (Report of the liver transplant at Kyushû Medical School used to promote the Brain Death Bill). *Shokun* 26(2):63–66.

Namihira, Emiko. 1988. *Nôshi, Zôki Ishoku, gan Kokuchi* (Brain death, organ transplants and truth telling about cancer). Tokyo: Fukubu Shoten.

Newsweek Nihon Han. 1993. "Zôki ishoku no saizensen" (The frontline in transplants), February 25. Japanese Edition.

Nihon Kyôkyô igakukai rinji kai. 1994. "Nôshi kanja e no taiô to nôshitai kara no zôki ishoku ni tsuite" (Concerning the management of brain dead patients and organ transplants from brain dead bodies). *Nichi kyûkyû ikai shi* 5:314–316.

Nudeshima, Jiro. 1991. *Nôshi, zôkiishoku to nihon shakai* (Brain death, organ transplants and Japanese society). Tokyo: Kôbundô.

Ohi, Gen, Tomonori Hasegawa, Hiroyuki Kumano, Ichiro Kai, Nobuyuki Takenaga, Yoshio Taguchi, Hiroshi Saito, and Tsunamasa Ino. 1986. Why Are Cadaveric Renal Transplants So Hard to Find in Japan? An Analysis of Economic and Attitudinal Aspects. *Health Policy* 6:269–278.

Perkins, Henry S., and Susan W. Tolle. 1992. Letter to the Editor. *New England Journal of Medicine* 326:1025.

Pyle, Kenneth. 1987. In Pursuit of a Grand Design: Nakasone Betwixt the Past and Future. *Journal of Japanese Studies* 13:243–270.

Sanner, Margareta. 1994. A Comparison of Public Attitudes toward Autopsy, Organ Donation and Anatomic Dissection. *JAMA* 271:284–288.

Sharp, Lesley. 1995. Organ Transplantation as a Transformative Experience: Anthropological Insights into the Restructuring of the Self. *Medical Anthropology Quarterly* 9:357–389.

Tachibana, Takashi. 1991. *Nôshi* (Brain Death). Tokyo: Nihon Hôsô Shuppan Kyôkai.

Tambiah, Stanley J. 1990. *Magic, Science, Religion and the Scope of Rationality*. Cambridge: Cambridge University Press.

Woss, Fleur. 1992. When Blossoms Fall: Japanese Attitudes towards Death and the Otherworld: Opinion Polls 1953–1987. In *Ideology and Practice in Modern Japan*, eds. R. Goodman and K. Refsing, 72–100. London: Routledge.

Yanagida, Kunio. 1994. Gisei—waga musuko, nôshi no jûichi nichi (Sacrifice—Our son and eleven days with brain death). *Bungeishunju* 72:144–162.

———. 1995. Nôshi, watakushi no teigen (Brain death, my proposal). *Bungeishunju* 73:164–179.

———. 1996. *Gisei*. Tokyo: Bungeishunjû.

SYDNEY A. HALPERN

3 Constructing Moral Boundaries

Public Discourse on Human Experimentation in Twentieth-Century America

DURING THE 1960s and 1970s, the treatment of human subjects in clinical research became an identified public problem. Medical journals published commentaries criticizing researchers for moral laxity. Newspapers carried stories of investigatory abuse. Congress convened hearings on questionable experimental practices, including exposing subjects to great risk without the possibility of benefit, drawing subjects from vulnerable—often institutionalized—groups, and failing to secure informed consent. Scholars in the newly consolidating field of bioethics articulated principles to guide investigatory conduct. Their standards enjoined researchers to avoid protocols involving undue risk, cease recruiting subjects from vulnerable groups, and obtain consent that is both freely given and fully informed. National commissions endorsed these bioethical principles. Federal agencies cited them in regulatory guidelines. Newswriters and academics invoked them in editorial commentary. Discourse in both public and professional arenas defined the problem of human-subjects abuse and recast the boundaries between acceptable and unacceptable investigatory conduct.

Among the noteworthy features of discourse on medical experimentation in the 1960s and 1970s is its disjunction with earlier treatments of human-subjects research. Although critics of investigatory abuse seldom commented on the discontinuities, in fact, the type of protocols they were depicting as ethically suspect had received quite different moral appraisal during the preceding two decades. Risk-laden nontherapeutic research was quite common in the United States during the 1940s and 1950s, and much of it involved institutionalized subjects (Advisory Commission on Human Radiation Experimentation [ACHRE] 1995; Harkness 1996; Lederer 1995; Rothman 1991). Far from criticizing such investigatory conduct, accounts of these experiments in the popular press typically celebrated the accomplishments of medical researchers.

How then did laudatory accounts of medical experimentation pervasive in the 1940s and 1950s give way to radically different narratives by the mid-1960s? To what degree did broader social currents affect contemporary moral discourse? This chapter examines shifting constructions of the morality of medical experimentation and the contextual factors that contribute to change. My analysis suggests that shifts in the culture at large strongly affect where the line is drawn between justifiable and unjustifiable medical research.

History is an especially auspicious site for exploring the social context of bioethics. In any given historical period, how moral options are framed appears inevitable. Boundaries between right and wrong are features of our common-sense notion of the world that operate as tacit social knowledge. But history—particularly history that refrains from imposing contemporary conceptual frameworks on the past—confronts us with the mutability of moral judgments.

Bioethical dilemmas often are framed so as to involve choices between highly valued but competing goals. Should life be extended or suffering relieved? Should scarce organs be allocated to the "worthy" or the underserved? Moral dilemmas in medical research involve tensions between the collective good that results from improved knowledge of disease and the well-being and rights of individual human subjects. How such dilemmas are depicted and resolved changes over time, in part because social forces alter perceptions of the nature and relative value of the competing goals to which moral choices are linked. Periodic shifts in the relative ranking of social goals inaugurate change in moral discourse. Thus, attention to human-subjects abuses in the late 1960s and 1970s occurred at a time when, as Deborah Stone (1987) observes, public health policy in general shifted its emphasis from promoting the collective good to protecting individual rights.

History not only underscores the mutability of moral judgments and their link to broader cultural currents; also it reveals processes through which change takes place. This chapter draws upon insights from the social science literature on constructionism to examine shifts in public discourse concerning research ethics. The analysis identifies several underlying processes. Contention and conflict surrounded public constructions of the moral character of medical research. Several groups endeavored to shape public discourse about the ethics of medical experimentation. For much of this century leaders of scientific medicine vied with regulatory activists—antivivisectionists in the early part of the century and bioethicists later on—to have its account of human-subjects research prevail. The ability of each group to influence public discourse rested upon its legitimacy, the resonance of its constructions with broader cultural imagery, and the group's access to arenas of public discourse. Although this chapter focuses on narratives on human experimentation, its constructionist approach may prove powerful for explaining developments in other areas of bioethics.

CHANGING DEPICTIONS OF MEDICAL RESEARCH

From the perspective of late-twentieth-century moral sensibilities, accounts of human experimentation appearing in the American popular press during the 1940s and 1950s were startlingly laudatory. Major newspapers and magazines ran stories on what would later be considered ethically unacceptable research: studies conducted on institutionalized populations and using protocols posing substantial risk to human subjects with no possibility of medical benefit. Reports reveal that medical investigators deliberately infected hundreds of prison inmates with potentially life-threatening diseases, including syphilis, malaria, and hepatitis. Far from criticizing contemporary research practices, writers for mainstream publications celebrated the contributions scientists and subjects were making to the public good.

Three themes in newspaper and magazine articles linked human experimentation to common social goals. First, media accounts underscored public health benefits resulting from even the most risk-laden medical experiments. These studies would provide knowledge invaluable for the prevention and treatment of serious disease. When a Philadelphia newspaper reported on experiments in which researchers infected subjects with hepatitis by having them ingest contaminated drinking water, its coverage stressed the importance of discovering that the disease could be water borne. The story included a detailed discussion of the adequacy of existing chlorination and filtration methods for ensuring the safety of public water supplies.[1]

Second, media accounts pointed to the necessity of human testing for the progress of medical research. In a *New York Times Magazine* article (13 April 1958), "Why Human 'Guinea Pigs' Volunteer," Alvin Shuster wrote, "the time comes, despite all the laboratory work, all experiments with animals and all the microscopic analysis, when only a human being can provide the true test."

Third, authors invoked contemporary cultural imagery in a way that linked human experimentation to the collective good. In the 1940s, this imagery concerned America's World-War-II mobilization; in the 1950s, its cold war goals. Press coverage in the mid-1940s of nontherapeutic experiments on infectious diseases routinely mentioned that the illnesses in question were a threat to American troops and that research was a contribution to the war effort. Pursuit of risk-laden protocols in the laboratory befitted the sacrifices of American soldiers on the battlefield: Human subjects were quoted in the *Reader's Digest* as declaring that participation in medical experiments was a way of doing something "for the men fighting overseas" (O'Hara 1948). The *Saturday Evening Post* called its 1949 article on streptomycin testing, "Are We Winning the War against TB?" (Potter 1949:34), and in a 1956 story by George Barrett, "Convicts to Get Cancer Injection," the *New York Times* referred to inmate-subjects as "test tube 'combatants' in the war on cancer" (Barrett, 23 May 1956). By the 1950s, some articles on human experimentation were making explicit reference to competition with the Soviet Union, such as Alvin Shuster's *New York Times Magazine* piece, "Why Human 'Guinea Pigs' Volunteer," which invoked the "race with Russia for space travel" and need for human experiments "before man can endeavor to embark on space flight" (13 April 1958). In the logic of wartime and cold war rhetoric, even life-threatening nontherapeutic research contributed importantly to the nation's goals. Human experimentation was an occasion for service to the community.

Media coverage during the wartime and postwar years by no means ignored the subjects of human experiments. Newspapers and magazines ran pieces focusing on the participants in medical experiments: prison inmates, conscientious objectors, and individuals "whose religious or other convictions lead them to such work" (Shuster 1958). These stories made a point of stressing the voluntariness of subjects' participation in medical research. The *Saturday Evening Post* titled a 1960 article on human subjects, "They Volunteer to Suffer" (Simon 1960). The *American Mercury* called its 1954 description of inmate-subjects, "Prisoners Who Volunteer, Blood, Flesh—and Their Lives" (Warton 1954). "Their lives" was an allusion to three deaths among prisoner-subjects during the previous two years that were mentioned in the *Mercury* article. It was the perceived voluntariness of subjects' participation, reassured journalists, that distinguished medical research in American penal institutions from World War II Nazi experiments. The *Saturday Evening Post* pointed to "the horrifying revelations of Nazi experiments on prisoners without consent, caution or regard for pain" (Simon 1960:87). In contrast, American researchers guarded individual rights by following a code of conduct "set down in 1949 following the Nürnberg war-crime trials" in which "voluntary consent of the human subject is absolutely essential" (Simon 1960:87).

Participation in medical experiments was not only voluntary, according to these accounts, also it provided convicts with opportunities for rehabilitation and moral redemption. Inmates, wrote Warton in the *American Mercury*, "welcome the chance to do something good to balance the harm they have done" (1954:55). And as an informant for the *Reader's Digest* concurred, "[Many] would do anything to redeem themselves in the eyes of mankind, and to bring some degree of pride back into their lives and into the lives of their families" (O'Hara 1948:35). "It's like the Boy Scout helping the old lady across the street" the *New York Times* ("3rd Convict Group Aids Cancer Test," 17 February1957) quoted one inmate-subject—the "street" in question being serious disease. Participating in nontherapeutic research was a chance to "bring the blessing of good health to others" (Simon 1960:88), to do "something not just for a few but for thousands . . . for generations of men and women to come" (O'Hara 1948:34). Warton wrote, "such projects boost the individual's morale enormously and give the entire institution a lift" (1954:55). And the convict-subject in O'Hara's *Reader's Digest* article agreed: "If I were in charge of penal reform, I'd install a human guinea pig ward in every prison in the country. I honestly believe it would be the greatest force for rehabilitation of prisoners ever set up—to say nothing of what it might do for medical research" (1948:34). The *New York Times* ("New Approach to Cancer," 24 May 1956) editorialized: "there is nothing but admiration for men who are regarded as enemies of society" and yet contribute to medicine "by willingly subjecting themselves to tests from which most men and women would shrink." In the public discourse of the 1940s and 1950s, there were no losers in the conduct of human experiments. Prisoners and conscientious objectors won moral redemption for their service to society; scientists received credit for strides in the battle against life-threatening illnesses; and the public was the beneficiary of important advances in the prevention and treatment of disease.

Celebration of nontherapeutic human-subjects research ended in the 1960s. By the middle of that decade, a dramatic shift took place in public discourse on human experimentation. Narratives about medical research invoked new language and imagery: exploitation of disadvantaged groups, unethical conduct on the part of researchers, unscrupulous practices by drug manufacturers, and corruption of public officials. The popular press identified a series of investigatory abuses: Jewish Chronic Disease Hospital, Willowbrook, and Tuskegee. Public discourse on human experimentation during this period included not only media accounts but also testimony presented at Congressional hearings (Subcommittee on Health 1973) and deliberations at government-sponsored commissions on the problem of human experimentation (U.S. National Commission 1978). Repudiation of existing investigatory practices reached a high pitch during the early 1970s in the aftermath of public discovery of the Tuskegee syphilis project, a study called "barbaric" on the floor of the U.S. Congress (Subcommittee on Health 1973:177). Journalists investigating prison-based drug testing reported "shocking physical abuses" and "a dominant pattern of human exploitation" (Subcommittee on Health 1973:797, 803).

Four themes recurred in published critiques of human experimentation during the late 1960s and 1970s. First, the selection of human subjects revealed serious social inequities. Researchers almost always drew their subjects from already disadvantaged and victimized groups. Journalists testifying at 1973 Congressional hearings insisted that "the earliest, riskiest and often shoddiest tests are conducted on the most helpless members of society—the poor, the retarded, the institutionalized" (Subcommittee on Health 1973:803). At Congressional hearings and national commissions, participants repeatedly returned to the issue of social inequality. "It is our moral responsibility," declared Senator Hubert Humphrey, "to see that the poor, the uneducated, and the captive are not left unprotected as human guinea pigs" (Subcommittee on Health 1973:179).

Second, critics implied that American scientists viewed human subjects as little more than experimental material. Many were impervious to the well-being of their subjects and willing to exploit those without power. In a 1973 repudiation of investigatory practices, author Jessica

Mitford attributed the following statement to a British physician: "One of the nicest American scientists I know was heard to say, 'Criminals in our penitentiaries are fine experimental material—and much cheaper than monkeys'" (1973:64).

Third, human experimentation in custodial facilities—where it was very often situated—bred corruption at both the top and bottom levels of the institutions. Journalists Aileen Adams and Geoffrey Cowan described arrangements whereby drug companies set up large-scale drug testing programs in state prisons. The institutions cooperated because of their desperate need for money. According to Adams and Cowan, "[O]nce they let drug investigators set up shop, large public institutions like prisons and mental homes seldom have the capacity to keep tabs on their work; and the enormous new flow of dollars into an impoverished setting has an almost unlimited capacity to corrupt those whom it touches. Wittingly or not, the institution has made a Faustian pact with would-be purveyors of medical progress" (Subcommittee on Health 1973:803). In 1972, the Associated Press ran a series of articles suggesting malfeasance among officials in the Florida prison system. Prison doctors and hospital supervisors were receiving thousands of dollars in payments from pharmaceutical companies to assist in tests conducted on inmates. This occurred "despite a state policy prohibiting prison system employees from accepting outside employment" (Subcommittee on Health 1973:872–878). Corruption associated with prison-based medical experiments was not limited to institutional officials. Convicts' involvement in drug testing programs contributed to vice among inmates. In Philadelphia's prison system, inmates working on a University of Pennsylvania testing project "frequently stole and sold drugs used in various experiments" (Adams and Cowan 1972:21). Furthermore, payments for participation in clinical trials allowed a prisoner to accumulate sufficient funds to "choose his cellmates and subvert them sexually with bribes" (Subcommittee on Health 1973:999). Inmate drug testing was linked to prison drug traffic and "forced homosexual encounters" (Adams and Cowan 1972:21).

Fourth, narratives of the late 1960s and 1970s rejected earlier constructions regarding the motivations of human subjects and the voluntariness of their participation in medical research. Critics insisted that many subjects never agreed to be part of medical experiments. Authors were especially likely to raise questions about subjects' willingness to participate when research involved critically ill patients, children, and the mentally retarded. Even where subjects understood the research and signed consent forms, the voluntariness of their participation was now questioned. Senator Hubert Humphrey, introducing a bill to establish a national human experimentation standards board, declared: "We have all personally experienced situations in which we were either subtly or overtly coerced into volunteering for something" (Subcommittee on Health 1973:177). Were subjects both fully informed about the risks of the research and free from coercion? This was unlikely if subjects were poor and uneducated. Individuals in these categories, Humphrey continued, "desperately need money and do not fully comprehend the danger to which they will be exposed" (Subcommittee on Health 1973:177). Nor were prisoners genuine volunteers. Critics now insisted that convicts were motivated not by the desire to serve society but by the money offered subjects, relief from the boredom of prison life, or hope of early release. "Can anyone honestly believe that there is a total absence of pressure . . . in cases involving prisoners serving extended sentences who volunteer for medical projects in the belief that they might get 'good time' before the parole board?" asked Humphrey (Subcommittee on Health 1973:178). Author Jessica Mitford raised the question more bluntly: "Are prisoners, stripped of their civil rights . . . free agents capable of exercising freedom of choice?" (1973:73). Mitford went on to suggest that medical research in American prisons was little better than Nazi experimentation (1973).

If public depictions of human experimentation changed radically in the mid-1960s, there were no comparable alterations in the character of medical research. Clinical studies that American researchers conducted during the 1960s and 1970s were no more hazardous for human subjects than experiments carried out in the late 1940s and 1950s. Nor were scientists more lax in their use of informed consent than investigators had been during World War II and the immediate postwar years. The total amount of human experimentation was certainly greater—a fact often mentioned in histories of American bioethics (Faden and Beauchamp 1986; Jonsen and Jameton 1995). The volume of all type of medical research grew in the final third of the century, a result of substantial increases in federal funding. But as discussed earlier, nontherapeutic research involving very significant risks to human subjects was quite common in the 1940s and 1950s. A number of the experiments identified as unethical during the late 1960s and 1970s had been ongoing for years and had generated no outcry when reported in professional and popular literatures during the 1940s, 1950s, and early 1960s. Why then did such marked change take place in public constructions of the morality of human experiments? Addressing this question requires examining the social processes through which public discourse is generated.

CONSTRUCTING PUBLIC NARRATIVES

A substantial social science literature exists on how social and moral problems come to be framed in public discourse. Much of this work adopts a theoretical approach known as constructionism. This perspective emphasizes that morally laden social issues are best conceived as the product of historical actors who deliberately strive to define what constitutes acceptable and unacceptable conduct. Howard Becker (1966) calls these actors "moral entrepreneurs" for the initiative they bring to the task of drawing moral boundaries and generating discourse that endows notions of right and wrong with the character of inevitability. Actors engaging in such definitional processes can be members of social movements, advocacy groups, and academic and professional specialties, or the leaders of organizations and institutions. Scholars note that how problems are framed evolves over time as does their salience as public issues. Hilgartner and Bosk (1988) identify multiple arenas that contribute to collective definitions of social and moral problems. These arenas include the press and other media, the courts, and the executive and legislative branches of government. Quite frequently, how a problem is framed is contested. Two or more parties formulate accounts of an issue and vie to have these narratives become dominant in public discourse. For example, advocates for labor and industry have struggled over diverse accounts of occupational safety, with labor insisting that worker protection is a moral problem and industry depicting it as a matter of economics (Hilgartner 1985).

Competing groups have vied also to shape the character of public discourse about human subjects research. For more than a century, scientists and regulatory activists struggled to define public images of human experimentation. Movements to control human subjects research went hand-in-hand with the emergence of modern medical science. The first regulatory activists were members of antivivisection (AV) societies that appeared in the United States beginning in the late nineteenth century. Best known for their objections to animal research, early antivivisectionists made human experimentation also a central focus of their efforts. AV advocates sought to discredit and regulate risk-laden nontherapeutic research. They were concerned particularly with research conducted on vulnerable groups: hospitalized patients, children (especially orphans), prisoners, soldiers, and paid subjects. Like modern-day ethicists, they questioned whether participation in medical research by individuals in these categories was voluntary. Antivivisectionists were the leading advocates for regulation of medical experimentation until the field of bioethics emerged in the 1960s.

Several things were at stake in the struggle between medical researchers and regulatory advocates—both antivivisectionists and bioethicists. Activists sought to redefine the boundaries between acceptable and unacceptable human experiments. Scientific leaders sought to legitimize ongoing investigatory practices. Activists sought to make human experimentation visible as a public problem and to bring about governmental oversight of clinical research. The research establishment sought to have experimentation viewed as unproblematic and to prevent government regulation of science. Each group promoted discourse consistent with its goals. Each generated its own narratives portraying the character of human experimentation—antivivisectionists in movement newsletters and treatises, ethicists in specialized scholarly literature, and scientists in publications issued by professional associations. Each endeavored to shape how human experimentation was depicted in public arenas, including the media.

Early AV activists sought—and often got—publicity for research abuses in the daily press. They expended considerable effort examining contemporary medical journals for evidence of objectionable experiments and then took stories of research abuses to sympathetic newspaper editors. Securing publicity for investigatory abuses helped activists advance their legislative agenda. In 1913, following sensational press accounts of research on hospital patients and institutionalized children, AV advocates persuaded legislators in Pennsylvania to introduce a bill that would curtail human experiments not directly related to the subjects' own medical treatment. The following year, U.S. senators sought support for legislation establishing a formal commission to investigate nontherapeutic experiments conducted in public hospitals. Legislators in New York and New Jersey introduced similar bills (Lederer 1995:87–89).

For their part, leaders of early twentieth-century American medical science mounted substantial efforts to forestall the movement for legislative controls. Prominent members of the medical establishment—William Welch, Dean of the Johns Hopkins Medical School; Simon Flexner, Scientific Director of the Rockefeller Institute for Medical Research; and William Keen, prominent surgeon and future president of the American Medical Association (AMA)—appeared before Congress and state legislatures testifying against government regulation. The AMA established a Council for Defense of Medical Research in 1908, which, under the direction of Walter Cannon, produced a series of pamphlets countering AV allegations.

Like AV advocates, scientists attempted also to affect the popular press. In the early decades of the century, Cannon contacted newspaper editors and publishers to influence the tenor of articles on medical experimentation (Benison 1970). At the Rockefeller Institute, targeted for antivivisectionist scrutiny, Peyton Rous, editor of the in-house scientific journal, instructed authors to revise their papers in ways that would decrease the likelihood of their triggering AV allegations. Rous advised authors to refer to research subjects as "human volunteers" and to substitute "test" for "experiment" (Lederer 1992:76). Early scientific leaders sought to avoid press coverage as much as shape its content. Through the early 1940s, they advised researchers to refrain from disclosing details of human experiments in scientific publications.

The research establishment changed its strategy for handling the press immediately after World War II. In 1946, it created a new organization, the National Society for Medical Research (NSMR), to promote the public image of human and animal experimentation. Among the society's goals was to educate the press—and through it, the public—about the methods used in clinical research. The NSMR flooded the media with information about the "how" of medical breakthroughs. This included an abundance of material on the rationale for human experiments. Among the organization's vehicles was a newsletter sent to one thousand science writers and a weekly "Research Report" offered to local radio stations. The NSMR educational policy was consistent with the strategy used by many scientific societies that, after the war, launched public relations campaigns to enhance public appreciation of science (Nelkin 1995).

Bioethicists pursued two strategies that affected public discourse. The first involved building a scholarly literature on the ethics of human experimentation. The initial publications in bioethics were written for professional and academic audiences. The often-cited 1966 exposé of investigatory practices written by Harvard anesthesiologist, Henry Beecher (1966), appeared in the *New England Journal of Medicine* and was directed toward medical researchers (Rothman 1987). But in the mid-1960s, leading medical journals were routine source materials for now professionalized science writers. Coverage of the issues Beecher and other academic insiders raised quickly diffused to the mainstream press. A second route for affecting public narratives was more direct. Bioethicists won appointments on federal commissions, established during the 1970s, addressing problems in medical research (Brock 1995). In this capacity, they formulated public discourse and reshaped the boundaries of morally acceptable investigatory conduct.

Shifts in public narratives over time reflect scientists' and activists' changing levels of success in affecting public portrayals of human experimentation. Regulatory activists were able to dominate public discourse in the late 1960s and 1970s; scientists in the 1940s and 1950s. In a still earlier period, neither group entirely prevailed; laudatory and critical accounts coexisted in the popular press during the early 1900s. The question of why social constructions of medical research changed over time resolves into two others. Why did scientists and activists experience varying degrees of success in influencing depictions of human experimentation over the course of the twentieth century? And why, ultimately, were bioethicists more effective in shaping both public narratives and moral boundaries than the AV advocates who preceded them?

WHY SOME ACCOUNTS BECOME DOMINANT

Shifts in the Legitimacy of Contending Parties

I argue that three dynamics contributed to the changing outcome of efforts by scientists and activists to shape public constructions of human experimentation. The first concerns the contending parties' legitimacy. During the twentieth century, discernible shifts took place in the prestige of medical science and in the status of regulatory movements. Researchers were best able to affect public discourse when the legitimacy of science was high and regulatory movements marginal. Activists wielded most influence when distrust of the professions grew and when critics of science included those in positions of social authority. Not surprisingly, trends in the standing of medical science and movements to regulate it were interrelated.

In the early decades of the twentieth century, medical science was still establishing an institutional foothold. Academic leaders were creating new careers in experimental medicine, reforming medical training to make it more scientifically rigorous, and pushing for the evaluation of medical therapies through systematic clinical research (Halpern 1987). The prestige of science as a whole rose with the advent of the Progressive movement and its celebration of scientific and professional expertise as a means of solving social problems. But while the legitimacy of medical science certainly was increasing, other currents in American culture also were at work. Some within the intelligentsia were uncomfortable with what they viewed as the impersonality and ethical insularity of modern professionalism. As science became the basis for professional standing, earlier notions of character, duty, and morality declined in importance (French 1975). Albert Leffingwell, a physician and moderate AV activist, viewed the willingness of doctors to use patients for experiments as an indication that commitment to science was replacing a tradition of medical beneficence. These changes, he believed, undermined the doctor-patient relationship (Lederer 1995). Such sentiments allowed the AV movement to wield substantial influence. The moderate AV position—favoring regulation rather than the elimination of human and animal research—received considerable support from within the middle and upper classes of American society. A wide range of professional and civil leaders—clerics, academics, physicians, lawyers, and even Supreme Court Justices—supported legislation introduced in the U.S. Congress in 1896 and 1900 to control animal research in the District of Columbia. In 1913, a hundred state representatives in Pennsylvania voted in favor of a bill to regulate nontherapeutic human experimentation (Lederer 1995:53). During this period, conflicting depictions of medical research appeared in the popular media. Scientists were able to forestall legislative controls, but neither they nor regulatory activists successfully dominated public discourse on human experimentation.

In the middle third of the century, when laudatory accounts prevailed, American medical science commanded an unprecedented level of cultural legitimacy (Starr 1982). Americans viewed science in general as an unequivocal asset, its aims fully compatible with national goals (LaFollette

1990). The standing of medical research benefited not only from the prestige of science overall but also from a series of significant therapeutic innovations originating in the laboratory. Medical investigators introduced insulin and sulfa drugs in the 1930s and antibiotics in the 1940s. By the 1950s, improved vaccines were controlling a host of serious childhood ailments. Researchers declared—and many among the lay public concurred—that medical science was conquering infectious disease. Meanwhile, regulatory movements declined in influence. AV societies had lost momentum during World War I and had remained ineffective in the 1920s. In the 1930s, activists reorganized and their advocacy continued through the 1940s and 1950s. But during the middle decades of the century, the movement was unable to recruit members or supporters from among professional or civic leaders. In the absence of broader support, it focused its legislative efforts on keeping lost house pets out of animal laboratories. Medical scientists made every effort to further marginalize the AV movement. Spokesmen for the research establishment dismissed AV advocates as a fringe element of vegetarians and kennel club overenthusiasts. Antivivisectionism was a "minor form of nitwit do-goodism" (National Society for Medical Research 1948:13).

If World War II was a time of unprecedented regard for medical science, the late 1960s and 1970s was a period of declining public trust. Articles appearing in scientific and professional journals remarked on the erosion in the standing of both the practicing and research branches of medicine (Burnham 1983; Ingelfinger 1976). Survey data further attest to the trend. Between 1966 and 1971 the percentage of Americans reporting "a great deal of confidence" in the leaders of the scientific community underwent a twenty-point fall (Etzioni and Nunn 1976:232). Public opinion regarding the leadership of medicine and a host of other major institutions underwent comparable declines (Lipset and Schneider 1983: 48–49). Meanwhile, the emerging field of bioethics inaugurated a new wave of regulatory activism. Both bioethics and early antivivisectionism appealed to professionals, including practicing physicians. But the new movement differed from the old in that its members primarily came from within academic medicine and from the ranks of other university disciplines. Cultural movements of the 1960s had made inroads within major academic institutions, including university medicine. The result was that a longstanding consensus within the research establishment concerning the conduct of risky experiments eroded. Dissent came not only from whistle-blowers such as Henry Beecher. By the early 1970s, rancorous disputes erupted on the editorial pages of the most prestigious medical journals—*Lancet* and *New England Journal of Medicine*—over the ethics of hazardous human experiments. For the first time in the history of American medical science, calls for the reform of investigatory practices were coming from within the research establishment. Medical scientists had lost both the cultural leverage and collective will to construct palliative accounts of hazardous medical research. The success of bioethics rested on both the legitimacy of the movement and the willingness of scientific leaders to accept redrawn moral boundaries in order to blunt pressures from outside and quell dissension from within.

Resonance with Broader Cultural Currents

A second dynamic affecting the success of activists and scientists in shaping public discourse is the resonance of their preferred narratives with themes in the broader culture. Historians have noted cycles of change in the character of American cultural and political ideology. Recurrent shifts take place in the relative primacy of liberal and conservative ideals and the relative salience of public purpose and private ends (Schlesinger 1986). These periodic shifts affect the ability of competing groups to influence moral discourse. Narratives are most potent and hold most appeal when their language and ideas echo themes in the culture at large (Gamson and Modigliani 1989). One dimension of ideological change concerns the relative priority of the collective good and individual rights. As suggested earlier, this feature of contemporary ideology is consequential for portrayals of medical experimentation because moral dilemmas in clinical research typically are understood to involve choices between the common good generated by improved control of disease and the rights and well-being of individual human subjects.

Not surprisingly, laudatory accounts of nontherapeutic research prevailed during a time of maximum emphasis on common social goals. Americans had a strong sense of shared mission during the period spanning the New Deal, World War II, and the early cold war years. David Rothman (1991) argues that World War II generated an ethos of utilitarianism that made nontherapeutic human experimentation acceptable. A broad range of citizens were making potentially life-threatening sacrifices in the national interest. Why should the human subjects in medical research be an exception? The change in public depictions of human experimentation in the mid-1960s coincided with a dramatic shift in America's cultural climate. In this period, radical social movements were generalizing the logic of civil rights to a range of other constituencies. The priority of collective goals gave way to concern with the rights of disadvantaged groups. Conflict over the war in Vietnam underscored the erosion of common national purpose. Public policy toward a range of health-related issues shifted from an emphasis on collective good to a focus on individual and victims' rights (Stone 1987).

The broader culture provided an environment favorable or unfavorable to the preferred narratives of scientists and activists. But the parties endeavoring to shape public discourse were not simply passive in the face of a hospitable or hostile ideological climate. Ann Swidler (1986) suggests that culture can be regarded as a "tool kit" of symbols and metaphors that actors can mobilize in the interest of achieving chosen social ends. Researchers and regulatory advocates actively promoted imagery consistent with prevailing cultural themes. In the 1940s and 1950s, scientists were successful at integrating broader cultural themes into public discourse on human experimentation: war against disease, laboratory as battlefield, victories of science, and courage and self-sacrifice of subjects. In subsequent years, activists were effective in promoting imagery dominant in the 1960s and 1970s: professionals abusing privilege, officials unworthy of trust, corporations exploiting the powerless, and victimized groups denied their rights. Language that, in this way, echoes broader cultural themes conveys a tacit but widely experienced sense of moral certainty.

Access to Arenas of Discourse

A third dynamic concerns access to influence over arenas of public discourse. The character of prevailing narratives rests in part on contending parties' ability to translate legitimacy into leverage over the ideas and language invoked by journalists, policymakers, and public commentators. Researchers and activists have been positioned differently to wield such influence, and their resources for doing so have changed over time. Not infrequently, contenders' success at affecting public discourse rested in part on alliances with powerful or well-situated third parties. The early AV movement was aided immeasurably in its efforts by the Hearst newspaper chain, which, well into the middle decades of the century, maintained an antivivisectionist editorial policy. Hearst papers were the principal source of sensational stories about investigatory abuse that stimulated support for AV legislation in the early 1900s. The bioethics movement of the 1960s benefited from the sponsorship of the legislative and executive branches of government, which, when human experimentation was becoming visible as a public problem, selected members of the emerging field to testify at Congressional hearings and to staff commissions on moral issues in human-subjects research. These appointments—based on bioethicists' credentials as scholars—provided direct access to crucial arenas of public policy and discourse.

The institutions and agencies serving as patrons of medical research were vital resources for the scientific community. During and immediately after World War II, the research establishment received help in its rhetorical efforts from the Department of Defense, which supported a good deal of the hazardous medical research being conducted by university-based scientists. Archival documents reveal that at least one Defense Department agency, the Army Epidemiology Board (AEB), actively intervened with reporters and editors to shape press coverage of nontherapeutic human experiments. The unit overseeing AEB investigations—the Army Surgeon General's Office (SGO)—routinely monitored press accounts of AEB-sponsored research. When objectionable press coverage appeared, Stanhope Bayne-Jones, the physician and colonel administering AEB research, launched an informal inquiry to discover the source of the information. He then sent letters reprimanding those responsible. The offending party might be a service corp member knowledgeable about AEB investigations, a university scientist receiving AEB funds, or even a research subject. Bayne-Jones found several unauthorized press accounts originating from conscientious objectors who served as human subjects as a form of alternative service.

Bayne-Jones put considerable effort also into intervening with the press. He corresponded with the science editor of the *New York Times*, sending scientific reprints and complimenting the paper on reportage the Defense Department judged to be "fair and balanced." On numerous occasions, Bayne-Jones allowed release of information to the press in exchange for the promise of editorial control over resulting articles. He would instruct AEB-funded researchers to cooperate with reporters if the newspapers in question agreed to submit their stories to the SGO for clearance. He then negotiated with editors over the tone and content of articles. He was particularly concerned with the language used in press coverage. Like Rous in earlier decades, Bayne-Jones took pains to promote use of the term, *volunteer*.

An editor at the Philadelphia *Evening Bulletin* wrote Bayne-Jones about a feature article on the "guinea pigs" in the "jaundice experiments on the University of Pennsylvania campus."[2] Bayne Jones responded: "Permission is granted for the preparation of this article provided the article is submitted to me for clearance through the Technical Information Division of The Surgeon General's Office prior to publication." The colonel continued: "It is hoped that in the preparation of this story the writer will maintain a moderate tone, and that exaggeration of the facts will be avoided. May I suggest that the term 'guinea pigs' for these *volunteers* is undignified, hackneyed, threadbare and hardly appropriate. I hope you can find a more fitting term for these men."[3] Pressure of this sort from an Army colonel with control over the release of valued information was bound to affect newspaper coverage.

HISTORICAL CONTEXT IN THE FRAMING OF MORAL ISSUES

The language employed in public depictions of bioethical issues invokes common-sense notions of right and wrong that are embedded in contemporary cultural imagery. Partly as a result of this, prevailing moral tenets give the appearance of being timeless and inevitable. But history reveals that neither the character of public discourse nor accompanying moral boundaries are fixed or inevitable. Constructions of bioethical issues shift over time as social actors vying to shape moral discourse exert varying degrees of influence over public language and imagery. Their successes and failures are shaped by the broader context: the ebb and flow of larger social, institutional, and cultural movements. These movements affect the legitimacy and cohesion of the contending parties, the character of rhetorically useful cultural imagery, and contenders' access to influence over arenas of public discourse.

This chapter has focused on changing constructions of the morality of human experimentation. But its analysis has relevance for other issues within the aegis of bioethics. One such issue immediately comes to mind: the moral status of abortion. Scholarship on the development of abortion debates (Ginsberg 1989; Luker 1984) shows that here, also, shifts have occurred over time in the character of the prevailing moral discourse.

Activists—in this case, of more than one ideological stripe—and professional groups have vied to shape public narratives and to define the boundaries of moral conduct. Again, competitors have paid particular attention to the use of language and imagery in the interests of moral suasion. And again, currents in the broader political culture have influenced the strength of the contending parties and the outcome of their rhetorical efforts. Debates about abortion and human experimentation have lasted for more than a century. Their trajectories make these issues auspicious sites for examining the impact of historical context on moral discourse and ethical boundaries. Many other issues in bioethics are more recent. As discourse concerning these moral dilemmas evolves over time, I expect that the dynamics discussed here will become increasingly relevant.

NOTES

Acknowledgment: Work for this chapter was supported by the National Endowment for the Humanities.

1. "Find Jaundice Carried by Contaminated Water," 12 August 1945, Philadelphia *Evening Bulletin* News Clipping Collection, Folder: Dr. Joseph Stokes Jr., Urban Archives, Temple University.

2. G. D. Fairbairn to Stanhope Bayne-Jones, 14 February 1945, National Archives, Record Group 112, Entry 31, Zone 1, Decimal 334, Box 676, Folder: Commission on Viral and Rickettsial Diseases: Jaundice Publications.

3. Stanhope Bayne-Jones to G. D. Fairbairn, 16 February 1945, National Archives, Record Group 112, Entry 31, Zone 1, Decimal 334, Box 676, Folder: Commission on Viral and Rickettsial Diseases: Jaundice Publications (emphasis added).

REFERENCES

Adams, Aileen, and Geoffrey Cowan. 1972. The Human Guinea Pig: How We Test Drugs. *World* (Dec. 5):20–24.

Advisory Commission on Human Radiation Experimentation. 1995. *Final Report.* Washington, DC: U.S. Government Printing Office.

Becker, Howard. 1966. *Outsiders.* New York: Free Press.

Beecher, Henry. 1966. Ethics and Clinical Research. *New England Journal of Medicine* 74:1354–1360.

Benison, Saul. 1970. In Defense of Medical Research. *Harvard Medical Alumni Bulletin* 44:16–23.

Brock, Dan W. 1995. Public Policy and Bioethics. *Encyclopedia of Bioethics* 4:2181–2187.

Burnham, John C. 1983. American Medicine's Golden Age: What Happened to It? *Science* 215:1474–1479.

Etzioni, Amitai, and Clyde Nunn. 1976. The Public Appreciation of Science in Contemporary America. In *Science and Its Public: The Changing Relationship*, eds. Gerald Holton and William Blanpied, 229–243. Boston: D. Reidel.

Faden, R. R., and T. L. Beauchamp. 1986. *History and Theory of Informed Consent.* New York: Oxford University Press.

French, Richard. 1975. *Antivivisection and Medical Science in Victorian England.* Princeton, NJ: Princeton University Press.

Gamson, William, and Andre Modigliani. 1989. Media Discourse and Public Opinion on Nuclear Power: A Constructionists Approach. *American Journal of Sociology* 95:1–37.

Ginsberg, Faye. 1989. *Contested Lives: The Abortion Debate in an American Community.* Berkeley: University of California Press.

Halpern, Sydney. 1987. Professional Schools in the American University: The Evolving Dilemma of Research and Practice. In *The Academic Profession: National, Disciplinary, and Institutional Settings,* ed. Burton R. Clark, 304–330. Berkeley: University of California Press.

Harkness, Jon A. 1996. *Research behind Bars: A History of Nontherapeutic Research in American Prisons.* Ph.D. Thesis, History of Science, University of Wisconsin, Madison.

Hilgartner, Stephen. 1985. The Language of Risk: Defining Occupational Safety. In *The Language of Risk: Conflicting Perspectives on Occupational Health,* ed. Dorothy Nelkin, 25–65. Beverly Hills, CA: Sage.

Hilgartner, Stephen, and Charles Bosk. 1988. The Rise and Fall of Social Problems: A Public Arenas Model. *American Journal of Sociology* 94:53–78.

Ingelfinger, F. J. 1976. Deprofessionalizing the Profession. *New England Journal of Medicine* 294:334–335.

Jonsen, Albert, and Andrew Jameton. 1995. History of Medical Ethics: The United States in the Twentieth Century. *Encyclopedia of Bioethics* 3:1616–1632.

LaFollette, Marcel C. 1990. *Making Science Our Own: Public Images of Science, 1910–1955.* Chicago: University of Chicago Press.

Lederer, Susan E. 1992. Political Animals: The Shaping of Biomedical Research Literature in Twentieth-Century America. *Isis* 83(1):61–79.

———. 1995. *Subjected to Science: Human Experimentation in America before the Second World War.* Baltimore, MD: Johns Hopkins University Press.

Lipset, Seymour M., and William Schneider. 1983. *The Confidence Gap.* New York: Free Press.

Luker, Kristin. 1984. *Abortion and the Politics of Motherhood.* Berkeley: University of California Press.

Mitford, Jessica. 1973. Research Behind Bars. *Atlantic Monthly* (Jan.):64–73.

National Society for Medical Research. 1948. *Bulletin of the National Society of Medical Research* 3(1):13.

Nelkin, Dorothy. 1995. *Selling Science.* New York: W. H. Freeman.

O'Hara, John L. 1948. The Most Unforgettable Character I've Met. *Reader's Digest* (May):30–35.

Potter, Robert D. 1949. Are We Winning the War against TB? *Saturday Evening Post* (Jan. 15):34.

Rothman, David J. 1987. Ethics and Human Experimentation: Henry Beecher Revisited. *New England Journal of Medicine* 317:1195–1199.

———. 1991. *Strangers at the Bedside: A History of How Law and Bioethics Transformed Medical Decision Making.* New York: Basic Books.

Schlesinger, Arthur M. Jr. 1986. *The Cycles of American History.* Boston: Houghton Mifflin.

Simon, Howard 1960. They Volunteer to Suffer. *Saturday Evening Post* (Mar. 26):33.

Starr, Paul. 1982. *The Social Transformation of American Medicine.* New York: Basic Books.

Stone, Deborah. 1987. The Resistible Rise of Preventive Medicine. In *Health Policy in Transition,* ed. Lawrence D. Brown, 103–128. Durham, NC: Duke University Press.

Subcommittee on Health, Committee on Labor and Public Welfare, United States Senate, Ninety-Third Congress. 1973. *Quality of Health Care—Human Experimentation,* 1973. Washington, DC: U.S. Government Printing Office.

Swidler, Ann. 1986. Culture in Action: Symbols and Strategies. *American Sociological Review* 51:273–286.

U.S. National Commission for the Protection of Human Subjects of Biomedical and Behavioral Research. 1978. *The Belmont Report: Ethical Principles and Guidelines for the Protection of Human Subjects of Research.* Washington, DC: U.S. Government Printing Office.

Warton, Don. 1954. Prisoners Who Volunteer, Blood, Flesh—and Their Lives. *American Mercury* (Dec.):51–55.

PETER CONRAD

4   Media Images, Genetics, and Culture

Potential Impacts of Reporting Scientific Findings on Bioethics

BIOETHICAL ISSUES generally are conceived of as arising within doctor-patient encounters and relating to matters such as the provision of medical information, decisions about treatment protocols, and the scientific investigation of treatment options. The vision of bioethics has focused largely on decision making, autonomy, and consent in treatment and research contexts. In this chapter, I want to broaden the scope of bioethics to include aspects of the social context that typically are not considered as "bioethical" concerns. Specifically, I will focus on how genetic findings are reported in the news and outline some implications for bioethics.

This chapter stems from research on how genetics is presented in the news. More specifically, my assistants and I are examining how findings related to behavioral genetics (alcoholism, homosexuality, depression and schizophrenia, violence, and intelligence) have been reported in five major newspapers and three newsmagazines, along with other print media, over a thirty-year period (1965–1995). The print press can be seen as an index of the news media; television and radio news tend to cover less science news in general and probably less genetics news as well. In addition to examining news articles, I have interviewed fifteen science reporters about their work. Data from this study are used to illustrate some ways in which presentations in the news media can affect bioethical issues.

SCIENCE IN THE NEWS

The news media are a critical vehicle for disseminating new scientific findings into the culture. The popular press has reported increasingly on science and health, both as part of general reportage and in special science and health sections (Klaidman 1991). Although the news media

90

report on only a very limited selection of the scientific findings published in professional journals (Conrad and Weinberg 1996; Houn et al. 1995), this coverage still accounts for a significant amount of information conveyed through the media. Science and health have become important "beats" for newspapers. The *New York Times*, for example, employs more than a dozen science and health reporters and publishes health and science news every day, frequently more than one article. Although there has been little specific research on how this dissemination of scientific knowledge is interpreted by readers, it is clear that the press is one of the most accessible means for transmitting new scientific and medical findings to the public.

Science and medical reporters tend to focus on a few professional journals, and these are overwhelmingly represented in the news: *Science, Nature, New England Journal of Medicine, Journal of the American Medical Association (JAMA), National Academy of Sciences, Nature Genetics,* and *Lancet.* Although other journals are reported occasionally, these journals dominate the medical-science news. For example, in a study of the press coverage of the association between alcohol and breast cancer over a thirteen-year period, 88 percent of the news stories came from studies reported in *JAMA* or the *New England Journal of Medicine* (Houn et al. 1995). These are among the most prestigious medical journals, according to science writers, and are the journals they monitor regularly. Reporters believe these particular journals usually publish the most consequential scientific research, and they presume the scientific findings are more likely to be of high quality because of their reputation for rigorous peer review. Although science reporters recognize that important research also is published elsewhere, it usually does not come across their radar screen. This narrow focus suggests that science reporting presents a very selective slice of biomedical research.

News science writing is not a straightforward process of "reporting" the facts of a study garnished with a few quotations from the researchers or other scientists. Science reporters, similar to other journalists, select, shape, and frame a story into news. Science and medical stories are difficult to present accurately and intelligibly to a lay public. Journalists often need to convert complex and ambiguous scientific findings into nontechnical, compelling, and readable stories. This requires reporters to simplify findings and to present them in ways that are comprehensible to a lay readership. A few studies have examined how medical science has been presented in the media. Dorothy Nelkin (1987) argues that science reporting tends to be uncritical and engages largely in "selling science" to the public. Medical-science newswriting often frames a story as "a new breakthrough in medicine" or depicts the newsworthiness of a story as "scientists report for the first time." There is some evidence that only studies with positive findings become news and that there is a bias against negative studies (Koren and Klein 1991). Negative studies and disconfirmations of previous findings are crucial to the development of scientific knowledge and are important to obtaining accurate scientific understanding, but they are less likely to be reported in the news.

THE NEW GENETICS

Genetics is a rising paradigm in medicine and science. People have long noted that some disorders "ran in families," and scientists have proffered hereditarian theories of various diseases, conditions, and behaviors. Eugenics was popular among scientists and lay people alike through the early part of this century (Kevles 1985), but it fell into disfavor because of the paucity of valid scientific evidence and the horrors of the Nazi genocide. With the discovery of the structure of DNA, a new genetics has emerged in recent decades. Along with producing some remarkable discoveries, the new genetics also has engendered fresh concerns about legal and ethical issues (Kevles and Hood 1992).

In recent decades, molecular biology and medical genetics have moved to the cutting edge of science. Important new discoveries, including genes for cystic fibrosis, Huntington's disease, Fragile X Syndrome, Duchenne muscular dystrophy, and types of breast and colon cancer, among others, have been reported in recent years. Many of these received widespread notice in the news media. The advent of the Human Genome Project in 1989, the largest biological project in history (Kevles 1992), has further fueled genetic research. The genome project is a fifteen-year, international research initiative with the goal of mapping the entire three billion base pairs of the human genetic structure. The avowed purpose of the genome project is to find the chemical or genetic basis for the four thousand or so genetic diseases that affect humans, as well as to discover genetic linkages to other diseases, with the ultimate hope of producing new preventions and cures. As the project proceeds, new claims about genetic associations and linkages with diseases, conditions, and behaviors will be forthcoming increasingly over the next decade.

The mapping of the human genome has been the object of several provocative metaphors, including a search for the "holy grail" (Gilbert 1992), investigating the "the essence of human life," and decoding "the book of life." The genome project itself has been called biology's equivalent to the World War II Manhattan Project. Others have suggested that the gene is becoming a cultural icon in American society (Nelkin and Lindee 1995), invested with almost mystical powers. Critics contend that the "geneticization" of human problems has expanded beyond scientific knowledge (Lippman 1992) and that a kind of "genetic fatalism"—assuming that a genetic association is deterministic and means a trait or behavior is unchangeable—underlies much public discourse about genetics (Alper and Beckwith 1993). What is clear is that genetic research is relevant to an increasing number of diseases, conditions, and behaviors, and that the genetic "frame" is becoming common for explaining a wider range of human problems.

An increasing amount of genetic research is appearing in the news (Conrad and Weinberg 1996; Nelkin and Lindee 1995; see also Condit, Ofulue, and Sheedy 1998). In 1995, for example, news articles reported research associating genetics with breast and colon cancer, diabetes, Alzheimer's disease, homosexuality, "novelty-seeking" personality, bedwetting, and obesity, among numerous other characteristics and conditions. Often these stories are highlighted on the front page of newspapers (including most of those mentioned above) because genetics seems to make good news. Stories about new findings are legion, so much so that it sometimes appears as if we are seeing announcements of "gene of the week" discoveries.

Although ethicists and others have raised issues concerning the potential harm of genetic screening and decision making, the privacy and confidentiality of genetic information, the prospect of genetic discrimination, the dangers of coercion, and the revival of eugenics (e.g., Bartels, LeRoy, and Caplan 1993), less attention has been paid to the effect of specific genetic information and the presence of new genetic and hereditary perspectives in the public sphere on bioethical issues. As noted above, the attempt here is to extend bioethical concerns into the cultural context by focusing on how scientific findings about genetics are presented in the news and examining some potential implications of these presentations.

In this chapter, I will examine briefly two science reporting issues that have bioethical implications, what I call the "disconfirmation dilemma" and the "one gene" issue. For each issue I will present two cases of genetic news presentations in some detail to illustrate the specifics of reporting and different facets of each issue. Although these are not bioethical concerns in the way that bioethics traditionally and narrowly has been conceived, they create a context in which bioethical dilemmas can arise and influence how they are framed.

The Disconfirmation Dilemma

Articles about significant new genetic research typically are reported in prominent places in newspapers or magazines. If subsequent research disconfirms or cannot replicate the first study's results, what kind of news coverage do the dissenting studies receive? This is an issue for science journalism I call the "disconfirmation dilemma," highlighting an information flow problem in the public discourse.

The Old Order Amish and a Gene for Manic Depression

In February 1987 major newspapers featured a page-one story reporting the discovery of a gene for manic-depressive illness. Based on research on extended families with a high incidence of the disorder among the Old Order Amish of Pennsylvania, a group with a stable and closed gene pool who kept good genealogical records, Janice Egeland and her colleagues (1987) identified a genetic marker that was linked to manic-depressive disorder. A genetic marker is a specific genetic pattern (or difference) found in individuals with the disorder; it is assumed the problematic gene is in the general vicinity of the marker. Although the actual gene was not isolated, the research depicted it as a dominant gene (i.e., it could be inherited from either parent) and pointed to its location (on the tip of the short arm of chromosome 11). The *New York Times* headline was "Defective Gene Tied to Form of Manic Depressive Illness." The news story announced a breakthrough finding: "Scientists have discovered the first proof that some cases of manic-depressive illness are linked to a specific gene defect" (*NYT*, 26 February 1987).[1]

A month later newspapers reported on an Israeli study of three large

Jewish families that linked another genetic marker (this time on the X chromosome) with the development of manic-depressive illness. The *New York Times* headline announced, "Second Genetic Defect Linked to Illness: Manic-Depressive Disorders Traced to Faulty Gene on X Chromosome" (19 March 1987).

Estimates suggest that two million Americans have manic-depressive illness. It has long been observed that the disorder has a propensity to run in families, and thus it was thought to be at least partly hereditary. The news articles sometimes offered new hope to people with the disorder and their families: "Once the faulty gene is identified, [Dr. Risch, one of the study's authors] added, physicians should be able to help guide high-risk people in developing a strategy for a satisfactory way of life. It might also help in devising a treatment that would minimize the risk of manic-depressive attacks, he said" (*NYT*, 19 March 1987).

Regardless of whether physicians can help guide individuals to more satisfying lives, even the discovery of a specific gene does not necessarily lead to successful forms of treatment. But these two studies presented strong scientific evidence linking genes to a susceptibility or predisposition for manic-depressive illness.

Two years later the Amish study was disconfirmed. In November 1989, scientists, including some from the original research team, published a paper that reported that continuing research among the Amish led them to conclude that the genetic marker probably was not significant in identifying manic-depressive illness. In one particularly important change, two subjects from the original study who did not have the chromosome 11 pattern and had shown no signs of mental disorder subsequently developed the illness. With the small sample size of these family pedigree studies, this shift invalidated the statistical significance of the study (Kelsoe et al. 1989).

To its credit, the *New York Times* reported this disconfirmation in the medical science section with the headline, "Scientists Now Doubt They Found Faulty Gene Linked to Mental Illness" (7 November 1989). Several other newspapers did not report the new disconfirming evidence at all or until years later as part of another article. The *Times* story outlined how the new study "cast serious doubt on the conclusions of [the first] study that linked a faulty gene to manic-depressive illness." It discussed the difficulty of assigning specific causes to complex and variable illnesses. The news story ended by noting that the Israeli study that linked a suspected gene on the X chromosome to manic-depressive illness "still seems to be unchallenged." In 1993, however, a research paper reported that after more exhaustive analysis of the Israeli data, the X chromosome link could not be confirmed. The *Times* reported this in a story in the health and medicine section with the headline, "Scientists Now Say They Can't Find a Gene for Manic-Depressive Illness," whereas three of the four other newspapers we studied never reported the disconfirmation. The *Times* story described how, in the wake of this disconfirmation and an additional one for a gene for schizophrenia on chromosome 5, scientists now believed that there is no single gene for mental disorders, but rather it is likely that the interplay of a number of genes with an individual's environment might produce a disorder. Again, the article ended on an upbeat note for genetics by quoting one of the study's authors: "Nevertheless, Dr. Baron remains optimistic that scientists will tease out the genes that go afoul in mental disease, if only they are meticulous in their hunt" (*NYT*, 13 January 1993).

Alcoholism and the Dopamine D_2 Receptor

A similar situation occurred with alcoholism and the dopamine D_2 receptor gene. In April 1990 *JAMA* published an article by Kenneth Blum, Ernest P. Noble, and associates (1990) that for the first time reported an allelic (specific gene) association with alcoholism. The authors found that, based on cadaver brain research with samples from alcoholics and nonalcoholics, "the presence of the A1 allele of the dopamine D_2 receptor (DRD$_2$) gene correctly classified 77% of alcoholics, and its absence classified 72% of nonalcoholics." The authors concluded they had found a marker for a specific gene in a specific location (q22-q23 region of chromosome 11) that "confers susceptibility to at least one form of alcoholism" (Blum et al. 1990:2055).

This study was reported widely in the news. All five major newspapers in my study sample reported the Blum–Noble findings on April 18, and all three newsmagazines reported it in the April 30 issue. The *New York Times* and the *Boston Globe* printed a story on page one; the other papers ran it in prominent locations as well (e.g., page 3). Headlines announced, "Alcoholism Is Linked to a Gene" (*WSJ*) and "Scientists Link Alcoholism to Gene Defect" (*BG*). The newspapers reported it as a major breakthrough. The *New York Times*, for example, wrote: "A gene that puts people at risk for becoming alcoholics has been identified for the first time" (30 April 1990). The newspaper stories were positive and optimistic, citing how this discovery strengthens the growing conviction that heredity plays a key role in alcoholism and that new drugs for alcoholism treatment could eventually emerge. The newsmagazines all reported the study, but were somewhat more temperate in their optimism. Although the news media did note some reservations about the study (e.g., sample size and unclear role of environment), the tenor of the reporting presented the discovery of a gene linked to alcoholism as a major breakthrough for medicine.

Eight months after publishing the Blum-Noble findings, *JAMA* published a study that essentially found no significant differences between alcoholics and controls (Bolos et al. 1990). The DRD_2 gene for alcoholism was not confirmed. This disconfirmation received some attention from the press, but much less than the Blum-Noble study. Although four of the five newspapers in our study carried some report of the disconfirmation, none of the newsmagazines did (Conrad and Weinberg 1996). The disconfirmation reports also were considerably shorter than those for the original study and were located in less prominent places (e.g., pages 20 and 59). Typical headlines were, "Researchers Cannot Confirm Link to Alcoholism" (*NYT*, 26 December 1990) and "A Disputed Study of Alcoholics Finds No Genetic Pattern" (*BG*, 26 December 1990). Although there was some reporting of the disconfirming study, often the stories were written in a manner that still affirmed a genetic basis for alcoholism. Both the *Times* and the *Boston Globe*, for example, quoted Blum as saying the gene was still relevant and that other studies supported their claim. An overall reading of the news coverage of these and related studies suggests the news media continued to emphasize a "genes cause alcoholism" frame in their reporting, despite contradictory evidence.

These two cases indicate that science reporting on genetics maintains a bias toward positive reports, suggesting genetic associations with behaviors or diseases. This is not surprising, given that others have reported that the media has a bias against negative stories (Koren and Klein 1991). In addition, genetic discoveries may pass for "good news" among all the bad news (e.g., crimes) and routine news (e.g., politics). But although the discoveries are trumpeted to the public with page-one stories, the disconfirmations are noted (if at all) in smaller back-page items. This kind of reporting is likely to convey the impression that a particular gene has been discovered, but it is unlikely to correct that view when disconfirmation occurs.

This of course is the logic of news: Finding something new is news, but not finding it may not be. Science is always provisional, however, so disconfirmations and modifications are to be expected as part of the scientific process, but such complexities do not always make good news. Moreover, newswriting often has to simplify to the extent that many of the scientific caveats or qualifications may be lost. And, it seems, the press considers discoveries to be important news, whereas disconfirmations are treated as inherently less important or interesting (or perhaps they believe the public takes that view). This approach parallels crime reporting: Arrests or indictments for crimes may be front-page news, but dismissals of charges or acquittals get far less attention and may be reported in back pages, if at all. Putative discoveries are news; their negation rarely is.

The "One Gene" Issue

News media use catch phrases to signify complex phenomena, such as Whitewater, Generation X, or tobacco wars. This practice is evident especially in headlines, but it permeates reporting as well. Genetic influences are complex, multifaceted, and indirect, yet news stories often portray genetic influence as if a single gene is responsible for a behavior or condition, be it a gay gene, breast cancer gene, or fat gene. This has been termed an OGOD assumption—one gene, one disease (Conrad 1999).

"Gay Genes"

Scientists and physicians have offered theories about a hereditary predisposition toward or the congenital nature of homosexuality for more than a century. In July 1993 Dean Hamer, a neurogeneticist at the National Institutes of Health, published an article in *Science* reporting the discovery of a genetic marker associated with homosexuality (Hamer et al. 1993). Hamer and his colleagues traced the family pedigrees of seventy-six homosexual men and found that 13.5 percent of brothers, 7.3 percent of maternal uncles, and 7.7 percent of maternal cousins were homosexual. They then conducted a DNA linkage analysis on forty pairs of gay brothers and found thirty-three pairs shared genetic markers on the Xq28 region of the X chromosome. Hamer and his colleagues concluded that "at least one subtype of male sexual orientation is genetically influenced" and inherited through the maternal line (1993:321).

Our research examined how five studies linking biology and homosexuality published between 1990 and 1993 were reported in the mainstream and gay press (Conrad and Markens forthcoming). Most received wide media attention, although the discussion here will be limited to Hamer's research because it is the only one to claim to have located a specific genetic marker.

Hamer's research was reported on the front page of five of the six newspapers we studied (we added the *San Francisco Chronicle* to our sample for reporting on homosexuality; the *Wall Street Journal* ran it on page B1). Three of the papers ran two stories on the study, typically one reporting the findings and a second focusing on reactions or potential implications. All three newsmagazines covered the story, including a nine-page cover story in *Newsweek.*

Hamer's research received detailed coverage in the newspapers. The lead in the page-one *Washington Post* (16 July 1993) story was typical: "Scientists at the National Institutes of Health have discovered evidence that some gay men have inherited one or more genes that predisposed them to being homosexual." This usually was followed by a more detailed description of the study and its findings. But for the first time, several articles began to use the term "gay gene" to describe the findings (even though Hamer explicitly noted that it is unlikely a single gene is responsible for homosexuality). For example, in three of the headlines, the term "gay gene" was used: "Research Points to Gay Gene" (*WSJ*) and "New Evidence of 'Gay Gene' in Some Men" and "Coming to Grips with Finding the Gay Gene" (*SFC*). In 1993 the *San Francisco Chronicle* was the only paper to use the term "gay gene" in both the headline and the article.

The gay press, at least as represented by the six gay newspapers we examined, reported Hamer's study. They gave this study more coverage than they had the previous studies, but relatively less attention than the mainstream press. Only one editorial used the term "gay gene," although other headlines implicitly referred to gay genes: "It's in the Genes" or "Gays with Designer Genes."

Within two years the term "gay gene" had become more common. When Hamer and a journalist coauthored a book about the research leading to the discovery of the Xq28 association with homosexuality, the subtitle was, "The Search for the Gay Gene and the Biology of Behavior," and the term "gay gene" frequently was used in the book (Hamer and Copeland 1994). When Hamer and his colleagues published a second study in 1995 (Hu et al. 1995), refining and replicating his research with a different sample, the news media again reported it. But now the term "gay gene" was common currency; headlines included, "Search for a Gay Gene" (*Time*, 12 June 1995:60); "New Evidence of a 'Gay Gene'" (*Time*, 13 November 1995:95); "Is There a 'Gay Gene'?" (*U.S. News and World Report*, 13 November 1995:93–94); "In Search of the Gay Gene" (*The Advocate*, 26 December 1995: cover); and "Study Provides New Evidence of 'Gay Gene'" (*BG*, 31 October 1995:1). Even a news item in *Science* had the headline, "NIH's 'Gay Gene' Study Questioned" (30 June 1995:1841). The writers also used the term "gay gene" much more frequently in the articles. David Miller (1995) notes that the U.K. press uses it regularly as well.

There are some stylistic issues worth noting here. On the one hand, it simply may be a journalistic shortcut to use the term "gay gene" instead of saying "marker for a gene for homosexuality"—it certainly has a more catchy sound to it. At the same time, the use of the term "gay gene" may indicate an increasing acceptance of the existence of genetic causes of homosexuality. Recall that both of Hamer's studies located only a section of the X chromosome (Xq28) that has a marker associated with homosexuality. At best, the researchers have discovered the approximate location where a "gay gene" might reside. It also makes a difference whether the term "gay gene" is set off in quotation marks. Putting it in quotes flags the point that it is merely a term that is in use (similar to saying, "so-called gay gene"). Omitting quotation marks suggests that there is such an entity—even though no such gene has yet been isolated.

It is also important to note that some writers designate it "a" gay gene, whereas others call it "the" gay gene. While neither is scientifically accurate, it seems to me the latter is more problematic. Hamer's studies are based on research of a very specialized sample of homosexual men: gay men who have brothers who are also gay and are willing to go public about it. Neither Hamer nor any other researcher claims that this or any other gene is likely to be "the" cause of homosexuality, yet calling it *the* gay gene suggests that it is the cause. Not all gay men have the Xq28 marker (probably most do not), so clearly there are other causes, be they environmental, psychological, or genetic (other genes).

And there is no evidence that whatever gene resides on Xq28 is deterministic: Is it still "the gay gene" if individuals who have it are not homosexual? At the very least, it is misleading to call it *the* gay gene. The more the news media use such terms, the wider the dissemination of the image of homosexuality as a genetically driven phenomenon, with all this implies.

There is a difference of opinion in the gay community about whether finding genetic links to homosexuality is good, bad, or irrelevant for gays. Some suggest that linking homosexuality to genes shows that homosexual orientation is "natural" and implies that gays should not be blamed, stigmatized, or discriminated against for an orientation that arises from their genetic makeup. Individuals who take this view argue that if the public understood a gay orientation to be an innate characteristic, such as skin color, then it would realize that gays deserve legal protection against discrimination. The T-shirt that proclaims, "Gay by Nature, Proud by Choice," represents this viewpoint. In contrast, some people in the gay community are less sanguine about the finding. They are concerned that finding a gene for homosexuality would lead to a remedicalization of homosexuality. Possible "treatments" for the "defect," such as testing fetuses and aborting fetuses with the implicated genes, and possibly even "eugenic" interventions (e.g., as depicted in the play, *Twilight of the Golds*) might follow. Others, including Peter Nardi, in his *Los Angeles Times* article, "Gays Should Lean on Justice, Not Science" (6 August 1993:B7), have suggested that because it is not sensible to base rights on biology, finding genes for homosexuality is irrelevant to justice.

Now the "gay gene" is more a social construction than a biological reality. Nevertheless, its designation may be having an impact on how we think about homosexual orientation and how we treat people who are gay.

BRCA1 AS THE BREAST CANCER GENE

Breast cancer is the most common cancer for women. It is usually estimated that one in eight women (12 percent) will contract it, and that forty-six thousand women in the United States die from it each year. In late 1990, Mary-Claire King of the University of California, Berkeley, announced that her lab had identified a marker for some forms of breast cancer located somewhere on the lower end of chromosome 17. This discovery was based on research on families that had multiple cases of breast (and ovarian) cancer (Hull et al. 1990). The genetic susceptibility for women in families prone to breast cancer is estimated to be strikingly high—perhaps ten to twenty times higher than for women without the susceptibility.

With this genetic signpost, a number of labs worldwide raced to identify the actual gene, now dubbed BRCA1. In fall 1994, Mark Skolnick and his colleagues at the University of Utah reported in *Science* that they had isolated BRCA1 (Miki et al. 1994). In a very unusual procedure, an announcement of the discovery was released three weeks before the publication date of the scientific journal article, in large part because of an *NBC News* report and persistent rumors of the impending discovery. On September 15, all major newspapers carried the story, most often on the front page. Headlines announced: "Gene for Inherited Form of Breast Cancer is Located" (*WP*); "Scientists Identify a Mutant Gene Tied to Hereditary Breast Cancer" (*NYT*); and "Scientists Say They've Found Gene that Causes Breast Cancer" (*WSJ*). The news stories were quite detailed, describing the BRCA1 gene as a tumor-suppressing gene, and circumscribing how this gene was implicated in only about half of all hereditary incidence and in perhaps only 5 percent of the total incidence of breast cancer. All women have the BRCA1 gene, but only a small percentage seem to have the mutated version that makes them more susceptible to breast cancer. For the women with the BRCA1 mutation, there is an 80 percent likelihood of getting breast cancer by age seventy and a 50 percent chance of developing it by age fifty. Natalie Angier of the *New York Times* pointed out that roughly six hundred thousand women carry the genetic defect.

This was unquestionably a major discovery, depicted by some scientists and reporters as a window to understanding all breast cancer. Early reports following the BRCA1 discovery implicated the gene only with inherited forms of breast cancer in highly susceptible families. Essentially, a defective BRCA1 gene was deemed to cause only a small proportion of all breast cancer. Yet if one examines the press coverage of this and subsequent findings, BRCA1 frequently is referred to as the breast cancer gene. Taking headlines as an indicator, we see many designations of it as "the" breast cancer gene, some appearing even before the actual discovery of the gene. A sampling: "The Breast Cancer Gene: A Women's Dilemma" (*Time*, 17 January 1994:1); "Vexing Pursuit of

Breast Cancer Gene" (*NYT*, 12 July 1994); "Breast Cancer Gene's Impact Limited" (*WP*, 20 September 1994); and "Return of the Breast Cancer Gene" (*Newsweek*, 13 November 1995:72).

It is important to note that although BRCA1 and the subsequently discovered BRCA2 (on chromosome 13) are genes linked to breast cancer, they account for a small percentage of all cases. BRCA1 explains roughly 5 percent of breast cancer, hardly sufficient to be deemed "the breast cancer gene." Research subsequent to the original BRCA1 report has suggested that a BRCA1 mutation may be more prevalent among Ashkenazi Jews (as high as one in one hundred compared with perhaps one in eight hundred) (Struewing et al. 1995), and that BRCA1 mutations have been found in some noninherited tumors. Yet even with these additional studies, it is probably most appropriate to call the mutated BRCA1 a gene that indicates a very high risk of breast cancer in women from families with a history of breast and ovarian cancer. It is important to keep in mind that 90 percent of breast cancer, at least at this point, appears to be noninherited. This is not to say that future scientific findings could not implicate BRCA1 or other mutations more widely in breast cancer, but current evidence does not warrant designating it *the* breast cancer gene.

Why should this apparent journalistic shorthand matter? In the most general sense, calling it *the* breast cancer gene (quotation marks are never used here) suggests that inherited genes are the main cause of breast cancer, which is not the case. Although the environment as a factor in breast cancer is discussed in both the scientific and news media articles, depiction of BRCA1 as the breast cancer gene nevertheless turns our attention away from environmental sources of breast cancer to germ-line DNA.

For bioethics, focusing on breast cancer genes raises a number of issues. First, calling a disease agent *the* breast cancer gene may lead women, understandably anxious about the disease, to request tests for the gene from their physicians. It is not clear what, if any, relevance the BRCA1 mutation has at this time for women without family histories of breast cancer. So far the gene's explanatory power is limited to high-risk families. Yet many other women will want to know they are free of the gene defect. Would a negative test lull women into a false sense of security about their risk for breast cancer, perhaps leading them to neglect breast self-exams or appropriate mammograms? Second, testing for

BRCA1 is an imperfect predictor. Some women in high-risk families who test positive for the gene defect may choose to undergo "prophylactic bilateral mastectomies," a radical operation removing both breasts, which still does not guarantee protection from breast cancer. Those who test negatively, although justifiably relieved, still carry at least an average risk for breast cancer, a one in eight lifetime prevalence. Third, even for high-risk families, locating the gene does not necessarily allow prediction of the course of the disease or lead directly to treatment. The gene for Huntington's disease, which was discovered several years ago, has had little clinical impact on that disorder so far.

In the near term, given the potential genetic testing market, it is likely that commercial products that allow for easy testing for BRCA genes will become readily available, according to Gina Kolata, in her *New York Times* article, "Breaking Ranks, Lab Offers Test to Assess Risk of Breast Cancer" (1 April 1996). Although virtually all the news articles noted that the discovery of the gene would have no immediate impact on treatment or even on prevention and detection, some were more optimistic about the implications. One reporter, for example, suggested that the discovery "sets the stage for a blood test, probably in a year or two, that would identify women who would benefit from intensive monitoring and preventive treatments" (*BG*, 15 May 1994). Another science writer was much more cautious, however: "Even when a test goes on the market, only a fraction of the women who believe they are members of families at high risk for breast or ovarian cancer should consider it" (*U.S. News and World Report*, 26 September 1994:78). This writer suggests that only women with two or more first-degree relatives (mother, daughter, sister) with breast or ovarian cancer or with multiple family members stricken with breast cancer before age forty should be tested when one becomes available.

More than a year after the discovery, Francis Collins, Director of the Center for Human Genome Research and himself a genetic researcher of breast cancer, suggested that for a variety of scientific, ethical, and social reasons, BRCA1 testing should be done only in the context of a research setting (Collins 1996). If "the breast cancer gene" becomes part of the common parlance, then many more people beyond those in high-risk families may want to be tested. Even putting aside the potential cost of unnecessary testing, what impact will a negative BRCA test have on women in a society where breast cancer risk is still so high?

It may someday turn out that BRCA1, BRCA2, and other genes yet to be discovered are parts of a collection of gene mutations that cause breast cancer. It is also possible that scientists will discover more specifically that genes and the environment interact in subtle ways to produce breast cancer or that some breast cancers are fundamentally environmental. As important as the discovery of the BRCA1 gene is, journalists and scientists should avoid simplistic designations that misinform and potentially misguide people about the risk of breast cancer.

IMPLICATIONS

Embedded in ways in which genetics is reported in the news is an array of issues with bioethics implications. This chapter has only begun to articulate these issues, but it seems clear that how problems are constructed in the culture and what is portrayed as common knowledge of them affect people's perceptions and what action they take. We can identify a number of specific issues.

1. GENETIC OPTIMISM AND RAISING PUBLIC EXPECTATIONS. Genetic associations with human behavior are reported regularly and prominently in the press (often on page one). The tone of this reporting reflects a genetic optimism, composed of the beliefs that genes causally are related to human behavior, that scientists will discover these relationships, and that these discoveries will lead to treatments or the reduction of suffering. The reporting of molecular biology and genetic associations tries to be upbeat and leave the reader with the idea that the discovery of genes is "good news." This is manifested in the ways the stories are written, notably when the last word in reports of disconfirmations is to the effect that better science or more research will yet find the elusive genes.

Genetic optimism resonates with the "magic bullet" conception of medicine—the faith that if we can just identify the right gene, science will come up with a biomedical treatment or cure for the disorder. Demands for genetic tests may increase, although their medical purpose remains questionable. As the discoveries of genetic linkages to Alzheimer's and Huntington's disease have shown, though, treatments do not necessarily follow from gene identifications. Genetic optimism, even when tempered by discussions of social implications (e.g., stigma or the potential loss of insurance) or by mention that genetic tests or treatments are not yet available, pervades the newsreporting of genetics. Despite these caveats, the tone of the reporting is likely to raise the public's expectations of what genetic discoveries will produce.

2. DISCONFIRMATIONS AND CULTURAL RESIDUES. Scientific findings are provisional and always subject to modification; failure to replicate results can lead to new understanding. The two disconfirmation examples presented (and to these one could add the discovery and disconfirmation of a gene for schizophrenia on chromosome 5 and several others) raise several issues about science reporting. Discoveries of genetic associations to common human problems are deemed important enough to become front-page news and are presented positively. They are infused into the culture. If subsequent research disconfirms a study, the press allocates far less space and attention to the contradictory findings, often completely ignoring them. This selectively creates a progenetic bias in the news and ultimately disseminates misinformation. The public is left with mistaken ideas about the relationships of genes to problems, and patients or families may become frustrated when the medical profession cannot deliver on the implicit promises.

The press's neglect of disconfirmations can produce errant cultural residues, obsolete ideas that remain part of public beliefs. For example, in the late 1960s the news media widely reported the putative relationship between the XYY chromosome and criminal behavior (Green 1985). This connection was disconfirmed in the 1970s. Yet when asked if they knew about XYY, some of my undergraduate students, who were not even born at the time of this controversy, replied, "Isn't that the criminal gene?" Without clear and proper reporting of disconfirmations, genetic misinformation may remain as a cultural residue. This may play a part in decision making around medical services as well as in shaping how society (e.g., employers or insurance companies) responds to particular disorders. Moreover, the fact that "successes" become news and "failures" do not reinforces the impression that genetics has more explanatory power than it actually possesses.

3. THE "ONE-GENE" MODEL AND THE OVERGENETICIZATION OF HUMAN PROBLEMS. When newsreporting uses terminological shortcuts such as "gay gene," "breast cancer gene," "obesity gene," or "thrill-seeking gene," it oversimplifies complex issues. These shorthand terms are especially common in headlines, but they appear frequently in news stories as well. They overgeneticize the issues they describe: Genes are depicted as if they were the most significant factor causing a phenomenon, when they

may be only a contributory piece. They convey the notion that single genes can cause diseases, which may be appropriate for cystic fibrosis and Huntington's disease (Alper 1996), but a single gene or OGOD model does not apply to most associations between genes and behavior or even between genes and diseases such as cancer. Calling a discovery "the breast cancer gene" suggests it is involved with most instances of breast cancer, whereas the genetic link actually explains only 5 percent of the illness. In other cases, such as homosexuality or alcoholism, no gene was ever isolated—only genetic markers were identified that suggest that genes probably are located nearby. Strictly speaking, there is no gay gene at this time.

In short, by terming a finding "the" gene, news media give the impression that genes are the primary cause of a phenomenon, which may not be the case. It privileges genetics in public discourse and reinforces "genetic essentialism" (Nelkin and Lindee 1995), that is, the view that human beings fundamentally are products of their DNA. In its extreme, this idea can become a type of "genetic fatalism," whereby genetic associations to behaviors or conditions are deemed to be deterministic and unchangeable (Alper and Beckwith 1993). Although unintended and unarticulated, this assumption could be the pessimistic result of geneticization.

4. GENETICIZATION AND THE SHIFT TO INDIVIDUAL RESPONSIBILITY. Implicating genes in behavior and diseases can influence attributions of responsibility for that conduct or condition. The locus of responsibility becomes the individual's DNA, and that responsibility has consequences. On the one hand, many in the gay community believe that if genes are associated with sexual orientation, they will not be "blamed" for their difference and laws will protect them from discrimination. If this is a valid argument—and there are those who would question it—what might a parallel argument mean for individuals and families suffering from alcoholism? On the other hand, when we deem breast cancer a "genetic disease," we shift responsibility for cause and prevention. If we regard genes as the primary cause, then we minimize attention to environmental insults that are associated with breast cancer and invest fewer resources in identifying environmental contributions to the disease. The woman (because of her genes) assumes responsibility for prevention, divesting chemical and environmental influences from causal responsibility. If the idea of breast cancer as a genetic disease gains common currency, it may affect how women engage in preventive behavior. Although genes may be "blamed" for the

disease, women are responsible for doing something about it. But even in cases where a BRCA1 mutation is identified, it is not clear what steps women can take to prevent the onset of the disease.

This shift in responsibility from society to the individual aligns with our current political climate, which increasingly blames individuals rather than social conditions for human problems. Thus genetics can become part of an ideological shift away from environmental and social analyses of problems, accelerating the decline of public responsibility for human misfortune and misery. To the extent that newsreporting privileges genetics in its coverage, it contributes to this shift.

Concluding Remarks

Whatever excellence is achieved in terms of the accuracy and clarity with which genetic information is presented, media coverage of genetics manifests journalistic conventions that frequently misrepresent the role of genetics in human behavior. News conventions, such as those pertaining to whether disconfirmations are reported and how findings are depicted, compromise the accuracy of science reporting. Perhaps inadvertently, the media reinforce simplistic notions of how genes affect behavior and contribute to disease and in turn affect public attitudes and engender new cultural myths about the role of genetics in explaining and addressing human problems (Conrad 1997).

In recent years we have observed at least one promising change in the reporting of genetics. Reporters, perhaps chastened by the prospect of disconfirmation, now frequently write that although a finding may be interesting and provocative, it still must be replicated by other studies. By the time Hamer's first study was published (1993), all the articles pointed out that these findings needed to be confirmed, and at least four specifically noted that scientific reports of genes for schizophrenia, manic depression, and alcoholism later had been discredited (LAT, BG, NYT, WP). This small change at least informs the public about the provisional nature of scientific findings and the need to be alert to replications and disconfirmations. It also will be important for the media to report on further research as it modifies important claims that have been widely reported.

All of these examples raise questions about how genetics has been "packaged" in the media and how that packaging affects what people think about issues and how they respond to problems, and, to a degree, what problems patients bring to physicians. Although in and of them-selves these are not usually seen as bioethical matters, it seems clear that they are part of the context in which bioethical matters emerge. By broadening the lens of bioethics, we can look for the sources of bioeth-ical issues "further upstream" (McKinlay 1994) and see their connec-tions to the depictions and knowledge that are common in the culture. One hopes in future years that bioethics expands its traditional concerns to include a bioethics of cultural information.

NOTE

Acknowledgments: This chapter was partially supported by a grant from the Ethical, Legal and Social Implications section of the Human Genome Project of the National Institutes of Health (1R55 HGO0849-01A1). The research assis-tance of Dana Weinberg, Nancy Martin, Ben Davidson, and Sarah Marin is gratefully acknowledged. My thanks to Diane Beeson, Barry Hoffmaster, and members of the Genetic Screening Study Group for comments on an earlier ver-sion of this paper.

1. The newspaper sample included the *New York Times (NYT)*, *Boston Globe (BG)*, *Washington Post (WP)*, *Wall Street Journal (WSJ)*, and *Los Angeles Times (LAT)*. For the subject of homosexuality only, the *San Francisco Chronicle (SFC)* was added.

REFERENCES

Alper, Joseph S. 1996. Genetic Complexity in Single Gene Diseases. *British Med-ical Journal* 312:196–197.

Alper, Joseph S., and Jonathan Beckwith. 1993. Genetic Fatalism and Social Pol-icy: The Implications of Behavior Genetics Research. *Yale Journal of Biology and Medicine* 66:511–524.

Bartels, Dianne M., Bonnie S. LeRoy, and Arthur L. Caplan, eds. 1993. *Genetic Counseling*. New York: Aldine De Gruyter.

Blum, Kenneth, Ernest P. Noble, Peter J. Sheridan et al. 1990. Allelic Association of Human Dopamine D_2 Receptor Gene and Alcoholism. *JAMA* 263: 2055–2060.

Bolos, A. M., M. Dean, S. Lucas-Derse et al. 1990. Population and Pedigree Stud-ies Reveal Lack of Association between the Dopamine D_2 Receptor Gene and Alcoholism. *JAMA* 264:3156–3160.

Collins, Francis S. 1996. BRCA1—Lots of Mutations, Lots of Dilemmas. *New England Journal of Medicine* 334:186–189.

Condit, Celeste M., Nnketa Ofulue, and Kristine M. Sheedy. 1998. Determinism and Mass Media Portrayals of Genetics. *American Journal of Human Genetics* 62:979–984.

Conrad, Peter. 1997. Public Eyes and Private Genes: Historical Frames, News Constructions, and Social Problems. *Social Problems* 44:139–154.

———. 1999. A Mirage of Genes. *Sociology of Health and Illness* 21:228–241.

Conrad, Peter, and Susan Markens. Forthcoming. Constructing the "Gay Gene" in the News: Optimism and Skepticism in the American and British. *Health*.

Conrad, Peter, and Dana Weinberg. 1996. Has the Gene for Alcoholism Been Discovered Three Times since 1980? A News Media Analysis. *Perspectives on Social Problems* 8:3–24.

Egeland, J. A., D. C. Garland, D. L. Pauls et al. 1987. Biploar Affective Disorders Linked to DNA Markers in Chromosome 11. *Nature* 325:783–787.

Gilbert, Walter. 1992. A Vision of the Grail. In *The Code of Codes*, eds. Daniel J. Kevles and Leroy Hood, 83–97. Cambridge, MA: Harvard University Press.

Green, Jeremy. 1985. Media Sensationalization and Science: The Case of the Criminal Chromosome. In *Expository Science: Forms and Functions of Popularization*, eds. Terry Shinn and Richard Whitley, 139–161. Boston: D. Reidel.

Hamer, Dean, and Peter Copeland. 1994. *The Science of Sexual Desire: The Search for the Gay Gene and the Biology of Behavior.* New York: Simon and Schuster.

Hamer, Dean, Stella Hu, Victoria L. Magnuson, and Angela M. L. Pattatucci. 1993. A Linkage between DNA Markers on the X Chromosome and Male Sexual Orientation. *Science* 261:321–327.

Houn, Florence, Mary A. Bober, Elmer E. Huerta et al. 1995. The Association between Alcohol and Breast Cancer: Popular Press Coverage of Research. *American Journal of Public Health* 85:1082–1086.

Hu, Stella, Angela M. L. Pattatucci, C. Peterson et al. 1995. Linkage between Sexual Orientation and ChromosomeXq28 in Males but not Females. *Nature Genetics* 11:248–256.

Hull, J. M., M. K. Lee, B. Newman et al. 1990. Linkage of Early-Onset Familial Breast Cancer to Chromosome 17q21. *Science* 250:1684–1689.

Kelsoe, John R., Edward I. Ginns, Janice A. Egeland et al. 1989. Re-evaluation of the Linkage Relationship between Chromosome 11p Loci and the Gene for Bipolar Affective Disorder in the Old Order Amish. *Nature* 342:238–242.

Kevles, Daniel J. 1985. *In the Name of Eugenics: Genetics and the Uses of Human Heredity.* Berkeley: University of California Press.

———. 1992. Out of Eugenics: The Historical Politics of the Human Genome. In *The Code of Codes*, eds. Daniel J. Kevles and Leroy Hood, 3–36. Cambridge, MA: Harvard University Press.

Kevles, Daniel J., and Leroy Hood, eds. 1992. *The Code of Codes.* Cambridge, MA: Harvard University Press.

Klaidman, Stephen. 1991. *Health in the Headlines.* New York: Oxford University Press.

Koren, Gideon, and Naomi Klein. 1991. Bias against Negative Studies in Newspaper Reports of Medical Research. *JAMA* 266:1824–1826.

Lippman, Abby. 1992. Led (Astray) by Genetic Maps: The Cartography of the Human Genome and Health Care. *Social Science and Medicine* 35:1469–1476.

McKinlay, John B. 1994. A Case for Refocusing further Upstream: The Political Economy of Illness. In *The Sociology of Health and Illness: Critical Perspectives*, eds. Peter Conrad and Rochelle Kern, 4th ed., 509–523. New York: St. Martin's.

Miki, Y., J. Swanson, D. Shattuck-Eidens et al. 1994. A Strong Candidate for Breast and Ovarian Cancer Susceptibility Gene BRCA1. *Science* 266:66–71.

Miller, David. 1995. Introducing the "Gay Gene": Media and Scientific Representations. *Public Understanding of Science* 4:269–284.

Nelkin, Dorothy. 1987. *Selling Science: How the Press Covers Science and Technology*. New York: W. H. Freeman.

Nelkin, Dorothy, and M. Susan Lindee. 1995. *The DNA Mystique: The Gene as a Cultural Icon*. New York: W. H. Freeman.

Struewing, J. P., D. Ableiovich, J. Peretz et al. 1995. The Carrier Frequency of the BRCA1 185delAG Mutation Is Approximately 1 Percent in Ashkenazi Jewish Individuals. *Nature Genetics* 11:198–200.

RENEE R. ANSPACH AND DIANE BEESON

5   Emotions in Medical and Moral Life

BOTH MEDICAL life and moral life evoke deep emotions. Merely contemplating a hospital conjures emotion-laden images: the grief of families of dying patients; the joy of new parents; the fear of patients hearing a diagnosis of cancer; the pride of a surgeon describing a technical feat; and the guilt of a medical student experiencing the first death of a patient. Moral life, too, evokes emotionally charged imagery: the vehemence of Dr. Jack Kevorkian as well as that of his opponents; the anger of demonstrators outside an abortion clinic; the anguish of a doctor on trial for having disconnected his own baby's respirator; and the public outrage at the suggestion that Mickey Mantle jumped the transplant queue. Such reactions signal that we feel strongly and care passionately about ethical issues, and such occurrences—both routine and extraordinary—tell us that emotions and bioethics are intertwined if not inseparable.

Yet although these moments are the very stuff of which moral choices are made, much of bioethics shows an indifference to or even a disdain toward matters of the heart. With a few notable exceptions, bioethics treats emotions in one of two ways. In one rendition, emotions are dismissed as irrelevant to ethical decisions. Insisting on a strict separation between facts and values and reason and emotion, an applied ethics model, as Hoffmaster (1994) noted, is grounded in a view of rationality that exiles emotions to the margins of its texts. In another rendition, emotions are viewed as barriers, obstacles, or impediments to "dispassionate" decision making. Because feelings subordinate the common good to the particularistic passions of special interest (Lutz 1988), they interfere with the disinterested objectivity that is taken to be crucial to moral decision making.

That emotions are antithetical to moral choice and moral judgment has long been a theme in moral philosophy. Writing some time ago, Bernard Williams, an eminent British philosopher, observed that moral philosophy has "found no essential place for the agent's emotions, except perhaps for recognizing them in one of their traditional roles as possible motives to backsliding, and thus potentially destructive of moral rationality and consistency" (1973:207). Williams cites several

112

reasons for the neglect of the emotions in moral philosophy, including the influence of "a deeply Kantian view of morality" (1973:207). Given that bioethics has been profoundly influenced by the Anglo-American moral philosophy Williams is discussing, and given that autonomy is a central notion in both bioethics and Kantian moral theory, it should come as no surprise that bioethics likewise has shunned the emotions.

Lest these remarks be taken as a caricature of one discipline by another, though, we should note that the social sciences also have been criticized for treating the emotions as peripheral. The current popularity of rational choice models of social action and the diffusion of "homoeconomicus" into other disciplines in the guise of the health belief model and the "free rider problem" in social movement theory are symptoms of this tendency. Some simplistic formulations of scientific method, still present in many social sciences, have promulgated the view of emotions as obstacles to scientific detachment and valid knowledge. As numerous writers have observed, social inquiry, like much of bioethics, is grounded in deeply entrenched dichotomies that divide reason and emotion, thought and feeling, cognition and affect, mind and body, objective and subjective, public and private, and male and female, inevitably subordinating the latter to the former.

But a growing chorus of voices in feminist theory, philosophy, anthropology, and sociology has begun to challenge the dualities that have held sway in the West since the seventeenth century, to reveal how social inquiry has been held hostage to them, and, with varying degrees of success, to transcend them. Those who write about emotions differ along several critical dimensions; they differ, for example, on whether the central phenomenon under study is "primary" emotional experience (e.g., Scheff and Retzinger 1991), actions performed on that experience (e.g., Hochschild 1983), or discourse about emotions (e.g., Lock 1993; Lutz 1988). Nevertheless, despite these substantial differences, it is possible to distill four key points on which most students of emotions agree.

1. EMOTIONS ARE A WAY OF KNOWING. In contrast to the dominant cultural and social scientific view of emotions as "irrational" obstacles to valid knowledge, emotions can themselves be a source of knowledge. The feminist theories of Chodorow (1978), Gilligan (1982), and Keller (1984) sought to loosen the grip of scientific detachment and a morality of abstract rules and individual autonomy by identifying a different (female) voice that is contextual, relational, and emotionally engaged, a voice that

can serve as a foundation for feminist morality and epistemology. Although these "cultural" feminists have been criticized for failing to transcend Western dichotomies and for promulgating a (cultural) essentialist notion of masculinity and femininity, they nevertheless brought emotions to the foreground of social inquiry. Hochschild (1983) called attention to the "signal function" of emotions in testing reality or learning about the social world, and Scheff and Retzinger (1991) noted that emotions provide clues to the nature of the social bond. Drawing on the work of Merleau-Ponty, anthropologists have identified emotions as part of an embodied knowledge of habits and practices that is often unspoken, tacit, and taken for granted (Gordon 1995; Lock 1993).

2. EMOTIONS ARE SOCIALLY AND CULTURALLY CONSTRUCTED. This point challenges the dominant folk and scientific view of emotions as private, presocial, instinctive responses (Jaggar 1989). Writers offer differing conceptions of the relation of emotions to culture and social arrangements. Jaggar (1989) and Hochschild (1983) emphasized the role of culture in creating "feeling rules," which indicate the emotions that are appropriate to given situations, and Hochschild (1983) showed how certain social groups are compelled to do "emotion work" to align their feelings with social expectations. Other writers emphasize the role of culture and social arrangements in shaping emotional experience itself. As Jaggar (1989: 135) noted, emotions "simultaneously are made possible and limited by the conceptual and linguistic resources of a society. . . . [T]he emotions that we experience reflect prevailing forms of social life. . . . [I]t is inconceivable that betrayal or indeed any distinctively human emotion could be experienced by a solitary individual." Finally, in a very different vein, both feminist theorists and anthropologists have explored "ethnopsychology"—how discourses on emotion are culturally variable and historically contingent (e.g., Bordo 1987; Jaggar 1989; Lutz 1988).

3. EMOTIONS ARE INELUCTABLY TIED TO POWER RELATIONS. Given the discursive dualisms that divide thought and emotions and subordinate the latter to the former, it is not surprising that attributions of emotions can serve as powerful tools for domination and social control. As Lutz argued, "[E]motion . . . becomes a residual category used to talk about deviations from the dominant definition of the sensible. . . . [W]hen the irrational is defined as emotional, it becomes sensible to label 'emotional' those who would be discounted" (1988:62). Although certain emotions, such as anger, are the exclusive prerogative of the powerful, emotionality is most

likely to be attributed to dominated groups in society, such as women, children, and the lower classes (Hochschild 1983; Lutz 1988). Not only have researchers explored how attributions of emotionality are used ideologically to disenfranchise and discredit, but they also have documented how the emotional experience of dominated groups is controlled more directly. In her study of hunger in Brazil, Nancy Scheper-Hughes (1992) showed how individual and collective experiences of bodily feelings are disciplined and controlled by larger political processes. The potential anger of the poor is neutralized as their bodily feelings of hunger are redefined as an emotional disorder to be treated with tranquilizers. It is also powerless groups in service occupations who are forced to do emotional labor, cheerfully tolerating abuse by customers in the service of management (Hochschild 1983).

4. EMOTIONS ARE FUNDAMENTAL INGREDIENTS OF MORAL LIFE. In contrast to the prevailing view of emotions as obstacles to rational moral choices, students of emotions have argued that emotions and values are inextricably intertwined. As Jaggar argues, it is no coincidence that many evaluative terms, such as "desirable," "admirable," or "despicable," are simultaneously words for emotions, and that we take pride in actions we evaluate positively and are ashamed of those we evaluate negatively. Indeed "the grain of important truth in emotivism is its recognition that values presuppose emotions to the extent that emotions provide the experiential basis for values. If we had no emotional responses to the world, it is inconceivable that we should ever come to value one state of affairs more highly than another" (Jaggar 1989:137).

In this chapter, we use these key points to examine the role of emotions in medical and moral life. Our analysis is grounded in our research experiences with two medical technologies: newborn intensive care and genetic testing. One of us (Anspach) has studied decision making in intensive care units for newborn infants. Neonatal intensive care has made it possible to save the lives of babies who would not have survived previously, some of whom have limited life spans or may survive with serious physical and mental disabilities. Consequently, physicians, nurses, and parents have made decisions about whether to save the lives of seriously ill newborns, decisions that have been contested legally and reported in the popular press in the United States (for more detailed discussions of these decisions, see Anspach 1987, 1989, 1993; Guillemin and Holmstrom 1986; Levin 1989).

The other author (Beeson) has spent more than two decades research-ing the psychosocial consequences of genetic testing. Some of Beeson's earliest work focused on women who underwent amniocentesis in the clinic of a large teaching hospital (Beeson 1984; Beeson and Golbus 1979, 1985). In this chapter, we draw also on data collected in a recent, large-scale study, in which Beeson participated, of families affected by genetic disorders prevalent among African Americans and European Ameri-cans: sickle cell disease and cystic fibrosis (CF), respectively.

Any effort to bring together information taken from several studies runs the risk of drawing generalizations that divorce observed phenom-ena from the local contexts that give them meaning. By the same token, however, when similar social processes can be discerned in three differ-ent research projects, we have reason to believe that these processes rep-resent recurrent patterns worthy of further attention.

The following pages are organized around three central arguments. First, many of what are ostensibly conflicts about moral principles are at their core conflicts over emotional experience and feeling rules. "Eth-ical dilemmas" also occur when an actor's moral precepts and actual emotional experience of moral problems collide. Second, emotional experience is shaped by cultural, social, and institutional arrangements. For example, medical organizations structure the emotional experi-ences of different occupational groups who work within them. Third, emotions both reflect and may be used to sustain relations of domina-tion and subordination.

Principles, Emotional Experience, and Feeling Rules

The ethical dilemma or quandary, a situation in which two contradic-tory moral principles hold sway, is bioethics' fundamental unit of analysis or even its raison d'être. For example, a physician's decision about removing a terminally ill patient in intractable pain from a respi-rator might be described as a choice between following the principle of preserving life, on the one hand, and the principle of nonmaleficence, or not doing harm, on the other.

Conflicts over Feeling Rules

Much more is implicated in such situations than a clash of principles, however. Indeed, many of what bioethics characterizes as conflicts over ethical principles are at their core conflicts over emotional experiences and moral precepts or emotion rules. Problems may arise when the emotions felt or displayed by one person violate what Hochschild calls "feeling rules" about the kinds of emotions deemed appropriate to particular situations. In the microcosm of the intensive care nursery, for example, a broadly based cultural prescription that parents should ceteris paribus love their children is translated into a concern with "bonding." The nursery's professionals have definite ideas about "appropriate" emotional attachment and expectations about how parents should feel about their babies. Usually parents are expected to become attached to or, in the parlance of the nursery, to "bond" with their babies. Drawing on the work of Klaus and Kennel (1976), nurses can view a failure to bond as a harbinger of child abuse. Conflicts may arise when parents fail to display the signs of "bonding": Nurses can view parents who fail to visit frequently or who seem to recoil from their babies with alarm.

Conversely, conflicts may also arise when parents become attached to babies with terrible prognoses or babies who are deformed or extremely unattractive—that is, babies who are seen as impossible to love. For example, trisomy 18, or the presence of an extra eighteenth chromosome, is considered in the nursery among the most devastating diagnoses: Most babies afflicted with this defect die within the first year of life, and the few who do survive are profoundly mentally retarded and unable to walk or talk. When interviewed about babies with trisomy 18, almost all of the physicians and nurses in both nurseries said these babies should be taken off the respirator. When asked, "What if the parents want the baby to live?" even those respondents who held that parents' wishes about treatment should be decisive now confronted a serious dilemma. An effort to probe the limits of respondents' commitment to this principle often elicited deeply rooted notions about "appropriate" and "inappropriate" emotional attachment. For example, when asked, "What if the parents had wanted the baby to live?" one nurse described the parents' decision as "inappropriate," because she didn't "think anybody wants to take home a severely retarded, severely deformed child." In such cases, the nurse argued that "you have to delve in deeper and find out why they want this baby" and that "there must be something else going on there when they subject themselves to that."

When confronted with the prospect of parents who want to take home a "severely retarded, severely deformed" baby, this nurse began to "delve in deeper" to propose psychological motives for what she saw as a clearly "inappropriate" decision. Similar reasoning operated in the case of Maria Sandoval, a three-month-old baby who had a chromosomal disorder, Rubinstein-Taybi syndrome, in which those affected are moderately to severely mentally retarded and also have physical abnormalities. The mother, a sixteen-year-old daughter of migrant farm workers who was receiving welfare, was asked to decide whether the baby should undergo surgery to correct a minor heart abnormality. What made this case striking to many members of the nursery, however, was not the baby's prognosis but that she was exceedingly physically unattractive: Her dark hair came together low on her forehead in a widow's peak, and she had sideburns and a beard. When asked what the baby was like, one nurse described her as "strange to look at" and noted that "a lot of people come in all the time to gawk and take pictures of her and people come from other places and other nurseries that have heard about her . . . and people making remarks, and other parents asking about the baby because she's so bizarre looking. She was very pathetic to look at."

The mother was told that Maria would die if she did not undergo the surgery, and she decided that the baby should be treated, even though she was not, in her words, "a perfect baby." But the mother's decision that her baby should be treated conflicted with the staff's feeling rules about the kinds of infants it is possible to love. In an ethics round in which the case was discussed, some physicians and nurses questioned the mother's decision:

Neonatology Fellow: I guess there were quite a few objections when she first came in, mainly from nursing.

Resident 1: I think anybody who looked at the baby has questions, you know, the radiologist we just talked to even in his casual encounter with the baby, was horrified (*laughter*). I mean both at her appearance and at the prognosis and what continuing medical care she seems to require. . . . And what's happened is that people have been sort of voicing their opinions that, ah, it's our tax money that is paying for some of this care . . . that's going to support this child in an institution, at some point that's what's going to happen, I think that's where—

R.A.: Which people?

Resident 2: Nurses.

Resident 3: I don't, I think I have a lot of those feelings. It did make me a little angry to see that kid and to think, you know, I don't have any desire to put a bag over her head, but I mean when it comes to do four major surgeries on the kid, I start wondering what are we doing? It really is, ah. . . .

Resident 2: It's also the resources up here, you know, if you're the one that's on call at night and she's sick and there's another small preemie and the residents here are limited, who should the care go to and are you utilizing your resources in the best available way?

Resident 3: I don't think it's hard to be interested in a baby, but I often wonder whether those same families would be interested when the kid's three year's old. . . . It doesn't take much to be a baby; it just makes me always wonder what the same families think when the kid gets toward one and is still doing the same thing.

"Horrified" and "shocked" at the baby's appearance, residents invoked a cost-benefit calculus, worrying about the resources spent on her care. When confronted with a mother who loved what they viewed as an unlovable baby, many challenged her decision and questioned her motives (see Anspach 1993), citing her age and her ability to know what was ahead. Because the Baby Doe controversies of the mid-1980s have changed the policies and practices in many U.S. nurseries, it is unlikely that professionals in today's intensive care nurseries would have contemplated withholding surgery from an infant with Rubinstein-Taybi syndrome. Nevertheless, the general point remains: In this case, the staff's conflict with the mother was clearly not about moral principles for, to be sure, most health professionals would repudiate the *principle* that an infant's appearance should influence his or her claim on life. Rather, the mother's decision and her attachment to Maria challenged the staff's deeply held feelings—in this case, about the kinds of babies it is appropriate to love.

Moral Dissonance

Although emotion rules and moral principles are distinct conceptually and empirically, they may, in fact, be closely related or may, in some instances, overlap when emotion rules are codified as moral principles. For example, the Biblical injunctions to love one's neighbor and not to covet are feeling rules that tell us that certain emotions are socially unacceptable. But most moral principles, such as thou shalt not kill or steal, concern action and enjoin us from acting on socially unacceptable feelings. People generally experience little conflict when their feelings and moral principles are in accord.

When lived emotional experience contradicts deeply held moral principles, however, a very painful kind of moral dissonance ensues, as the following case suggests:

> A Catholic woman, who believes strongly that abortion is morally wrong, was devastated to learn that her infant son had CF. Three years later she learned that she had accidentally become pregnant. Having observed her first son's suffering, she could not accept the possibility of giving birth to another child who would be afflicted with the same disease, and she chose to violate her own principles by having an abortion. The result of this dissonance was intense shame and guilt. When she came to this point in describing her reproductive history, she lowered her voice and whispered, "I don't like talking about it, but in between I did abort one because there was nothing they could do for me at that point." This is a reference to the fact that prenatal testing for CF was not yet available. She adds, "I feel very guilty about it." Later, she became pregnant a third time because she was told prenatal diagnosis for CF had become available. The results of the test were inconclusive, however. Still feeling guilty about the previous abortion, she continued the pregnancy: "I just said I was not going to go through that again."

With each pregnancy after her son's diagnosis, this woman's dissonance between her lived emotional experience with CF and her moral principles produced a different, but ultimately unsatisfactory, resolution. When she became pregnant for the second time, she resolved the dissonance between her antiabortion principles and her painful emotional experience with a child with CF by completely revising her moral stance and choosing abortion for CF—only to experience subsequent shame and guilt. The third pregnancy produced metaemotion (in this case, the woman's anticipatory fear of guilt), which guided her moral choice to continue a pregnancy that occurred only because she believed prenatal testing would enable her to prevent the birth of another affected child. But her dread of another abortion had a signal function, because it told her she could not live with the burden of yet another violation of her moral precepts.

Ethical theories provide for the rational dissonance that results from a conflict between two principles, and social psychologists identify the cognitive dissonance that results from conflicting beliefs. Hochschild (1983:90) identifies still another kind of dissonance—emotive dissonance—that occurs when emotional experience violates feeling rules. But the intense inner conflict experienced by the woman in the previous case represents yet another dissonance not captured by the concepts just described. This fourth kind of dissonance, which we call moral dissonance, represents a deep disjuncture between the emotional and the moral realms. In this case the woman's moral dissonance occurred when lived emotional experience and the moral order collided.

As this case suggests, moral dissonance might also result when, for a variety of reasons, people are forced to act in ways that contradict their moral principles. This type of dissonance occurs frequently in the newborn intensive care unit. Neonatal intensive care is committed to improving the care of critically ill newborns, both in terms of their survival and in terms of their quality of life (mortality and morbidity). But given that mortality decreases much faster than morbidity, the number of infants with serious mental and physical disabilities is increasing. This pattern holds particularly for the smallest premature infants—infants who weigh as little as one pound—who now survive because of neonatology's advances (for discussions of these issues, see, for example, Budetti et al. 1980; Stewart 1989). So morbidity continues to be a fact of life in today's intensive care nurseries, and this means that, at one time or another, professionals in the nursery must care for the occasional baby who is likely to survive with serious disabilities (e.g., blindness, cerebral palsy, severe mental retardation) and who is alive because of their own medical interventions. Caring for a tiny premature infant who displays the first signs of cerebral palsy or a badly asphyxiated infant whose seizures cannot be controlled threatens the very foundation of the neonatal enterprise, for these experiences force professionals to face their own violations of their primary moral injunction to do no harm. The result of the ensuing dissonance can be depression or guilt.

Nursery staff members have developed strategies to cope with dissonance between their moral vision of the enterprise and their actions. There are, first, the collections of words, props, habits, and practices that transform a patient from a person with a past and a future into a docile object or collection of body parts. The screen that separates the patient's face and body during surgery has a counterpart in the depersonalizing language of case presentations that separates biological processes from their owners ("the lungs" not "his lungs," "the pregnancy" not "her pregnancy"). Such practices can allow professionals to keep problematic emotions at bay (for discussions of these issues, see Anspach 1988; Chambliss 1996; Hochschild 1983). One collective coping mechanism apparent to any visitor to the nursery is many photos and postcards from grateful parents that are posted on a bulletin board. Collective rituals of validation are yet another means of reducing moral dissonance. For example, every year staff hold a Christmas party for "graduates of the nursery"— and, needless to say, only happy, grateful parents are likely to attend. Of course, attending neonatologists can avoid much of this dissonance by simply adopting the experimental article of faith that the health of some of today's survivors is the inevitable price of progress, a necessary sacrifice for tomorrow's infants (for a discussion of this issue, see Fox and Swazey 1984). Those who are most likely to experience dissonance between principles and action are the nurses, who, having little power, are forced to care for the babies others have decided to save. Despite the increasing professionalization of the nursing profession, nursing ethics, Chambliss observes, remain the ethics of the quintessentially powerless: "Devoutly prolife nurses may be asked to let deformed infants die, to disconnect ventilators. They must often carry out policies they deplore, orders they believe wrong, and treatments they believe are cruel" (Chambliss 1996:87–88). In such instances of moral dissonance, the emotional experiences of professionals are shaped by their location in a bureaucratic structure, an issue we now explore.

INSTITUTIONAL ARRANGEMENTS AND EMOTIONAL EXPERIENCE: ETHICS OF ENGAGEMENT AND DETACHMENT

Physicians and Nurses

Emotional experience is not, as conventional wisdom would have us believe, exclusively a private, individual matter; rather, it is shaped by social and institutional arrangements. The organization of the newborn intensive care unit, for instance, structures the emotional experiences of those who work within it, leading to conflicting views of the right thing to do. Perhaps the most compelling example of how the intensive care nursery generates such conflicts is the clash between the nurses' embodied ethics of engagement and the physicians' ethic of emotional detachment. The nurses' continuous contact and interaction with infants and parents leads to emotional engagement and fosters the development of emotions—both positive and negative.[1] The contact of physicians with patients and families is, in contrast, limited and technically focused. The greater structural engagement of the nurses can lead them to have a heightened sense of their patients' suffering that can propel them into intense conflicts with physicians, particularly in situations where treatment is viewed as experimental:

> Roberta Zapata, the ninth child of farm workers, was diagnosed as having an arteriovenous malformation in the vein of Galen (an abnormal connection between a vein and an artery in the brain). Roberta was referred to the nursery, where a neurosurgeon had developed an operation that involved inserting fifty feet of fine wire into the malformation to induce a blood clot that would close the malformation. This operation, which this neurosurgeon had performed successfully on adults and older children, had never before been attempted on an infant. Altogether Roberta underwent four operations: the first two involved inserting wire into the malformation, and the third and fourth operations were performed to clip off the blood vessels that fed into the lesion. Roberta returned from the third operation seizing violently. At this point, the nurses voiced strong objections to performing another operation. In the eyes of many nurses, Roberta had "become an experimental animal for the neurosurgeons":

>> They had no feeling for her suffering as a person. They don't sit here and watch her day and night. One night she was having convulsions and her head was leaking cerebrospinal fluid all over, so we called the neurosurgeon. He came in and bandaged her head, and I mean he scrubbed her head with betadyne. Now I grant you she had an infection, but it was the way he did, like you would scrub a table, and then we said, "why don't you give her some xylocaine?" and he said, "oh no," and stitched up her head without anesthesia. This is what made us angry; she's not a person to them, she's just their experiment.

> Despite the objections of the nurses, the neurosurgeons operated once again, and only after the fourth surgery did they agree that no further operations were to be performed. Roberta finally died of meningitis, which was not treated.

The disagreement in this case perhaps derives from differing concepts of "success" or different resolutions of the experiment–therapy dilemma, which forces physicians to balance eagerness to advance knowledge against possible harm to the patient being treated. For the physicians interviewed after Roberta had died, the operations were not a failure. They had seen some improvement in decreasing the size of the lesion, and they had stopped only when no further gains were to be made and the operations could not advance the care of other patients in the future. For the nurses who sat at the bedside, Roberta was a suffering, sentient person, and the procedures were far from successful. As is often true in a teaching hospital, the nurses accused the physicians of sacrificing matters of the heart on the altar of scientific zeal. This was particularly likely when the physicians were specialists, outsiders to the nursery, who, from the nurses' perspective, could be insulated from the consequences of their actions and inured to the suffering of their patients.

While nurses' structural engagement can lead to greater emotional engagement, continuous contact with infants also has its shadow side, permitting negative emotions—as well as empathy—to flourish. Thus, it is not uncommon to hear nurses talk about "hating" to take care of babies who are unattractive, who are unresponsive or negatively responsive, or who require chronic care—infants who provide few rewards and are difficult to manage. Recall that with Maria Sandoval residents reported that it was the nurses who objected most strenuously to the operation. This pattern was confirmed by interviews in which nurses spoke of being repelled by her appearance and, moreover, found her difficult to feed. Although no nurse would view these factors in themselves as sufficient grounds for withholding surgery, when combined with a prognosis of mental retardation and a heart defect, they led some nurses to question the baby's future quality of life:

> I felt real strongly about that baby not going to have a PDA ligation [a procedure to correct patent ductus arteriosis, a heart defect], and that was the mother's decision, and I don't know if she realized what all this entailed, what the baby was going to go through, what she was going to go through. . . . [R.A.: What should a parent like this be told?] The prognosis is not very good. . . . Their IQ's are very low; they're able to do very little, possibly feed themselves; and their general appearance is very gross too, and that's not going to help anybody in this society, help the kid at all.

More commonly, nurses' feelings about Maria Sandoval's appearance and their difficulties caring for her created an overall gestalt that tacitly colored their views of her prognosis This becomes apparent when we contrast their views of Maria with their views of an infant with Down syndrome. Both babies have similar prognoses, and both need surgical procedures that are relatively easy to perform. The only distinction between the two babies is that Maria was unattractive and posed management problems. Almost all of the nurses (but few residents) who had taken care of Maria viewed her prognosis as significantly worse than that of a baby with Down syndrome:

R.A.: How does this baby compare to a Down's?

R.: It's worse than a Down's.

R.A.: In what way?

R.: In that the amount of retardation is more severe than a Down's. A lot of Down's are able to exist outside of institutions, a lot aren't—but they still have classes that these kids can be in—they're trainable, whereas a Rubinstein just doesn't seem to be trainable with such a low IQ.

By contrast, those nurses who had not seen the baby perceived her intellectual potential as equivalent to that of a baby with Down syndrome. Nurses' greater structural and emotional engagement is, then, a double-edged sword. It can, on the one hand, provide the social foundations for empathy and a heightened awareness of patients as persons who suffer. On the other hand, continuous contact can lead nurses to adopt negative attitudes toward infants who provide few rewards or who pose management problems.

This is not to say, however, that the physician's perspective, the ethics of detachment, is better or more "true," for emotional detachment is also a double-edged sword. The two-sidedness of detachment is apparent in definitions of the word "objective," which means both free from personal bias and impartial as well as treating the other as an object. Clinical detachment, as Zussman (1992) notes, can lead physicians to treat all patients equally as objects of medical intervention and, in this sense, can protect patients from discrimination. But detachment produces a limited kind of justice, a narrow bureaucratic rationality. (Recall that for Weber [1946] "without regard for persons" is the watchword of bureaucracy.) A perspective that filters out the personal, the emotional, is a limited angle of vision indeed. For just as the nurses' perspective may be colored by their frustrations in caring for infants who pose management problems, so, too, physicians' structural and emotional detachment from patients and families (coupled with a possible investment in learning something from the case) may blind them to suffering and propel them into highly aggressive lines of action.

Parents and Emotional Engagement

Despite the differences between physicians and nurses that we have discussed, all professionals participate in a culture that routinizes pain and death and in practices that transform patients into collections of body parts or objects (Chambliss 1996). For this reason, conflicts between parents and professionals (including nurses) can arise out of the greater engagement and attachment that often develops between parents and their babies, as occurred with Maria Sandoval.

As the reactions to Maria Sandoval show, the different emotional contexts of parent-child relationships and staff-child relationships may lead to conflicts about life-and-death decisions. Thus, babies with trisomy 13 (an extra thirteenth chromosome) and trisomy 18 (an extra eighteenth chromosome) have a similar prognosis: a short life expectancy and severe mental retardation. These infants, however, actually appear very different. Whereas infants with trisomy 13 are often grossly malformed, infants with trisomy 18 may look like "normal" babies. For this reason, some parents of infants with trisomy 18 may become attached to them and may even question the grim prognosis presented by staff (for a discussion of this issue, see Anspach 1993:134–135).

In some cases, parents' greater attachment to their babies may lead them to challenge staff decisions to perform procedures that the parents feel will cause their babies pain and suffering, but that professionals view as routine. One nurse, whose baby had been hospitalized in an intensive care unit, commented: "Coming in and finding a Band-Aid on our baby's foot or a bruise on his head, what that must mean to a parent, we take for granted because we see it all the time. But when you come in, that may be the hugest thing a parent notices, this huge bruise on his head. It's routine, but not for a parent."

Conflicts can also occur in the opposite direction because medical technologies can cause parents to disengage emotionally. In a study of couples undergoing prenatal diagnosis for Down syndrome and other chromosomal disorders, Beeson (Beeson 1984; Beeson and Golbus 1979) identified a phenomenon she called "suspension of commitment to pregnancy." This strategy is employed by women and their partners to cope with the threat that the pregnancy might not result in a healthy child. It consists of hiding the physical changes of pregnancy, not wearing maternity clothes, and keeping the pregnancy secret. (For a related discussion, see Rothman 1986.) This strategy protected expectant mothers from constant reminders of the uncertainties about whether they would continue the pregnancy. It also protected them from the emotional discomfort of having to acknowledge publicly an unfavorable result and an ensuing abortion, should these events occur, while at the same time enabling pregnant women to protect extended family members—particularly parents—from a possible sense of loss.

Suspension of commitment to pregnancy is a strategy that involves considerable "emotion work," to use Hochschild's (1983) term. Many women worked very deliberately to keep their attention focused on projects unrelated to the pregnancy during the weeks they waited for test results. In some cases, this led to difficulties in gaining weight, stopping smoking, or taking prenatal vitamins. Beeson (1984) noted some class variation in the type and extent of emotion work involved in suspending commitment to pregnancy. For most women and their partners, however, a telephone call from the clinic announcing favorable laboratory results immediately transforms emotional detachment into more intense and usually joyful engagement in the pregnancy. At this point, when parents usually learn both the test results and the sex of their future child, naming often takes place.

Just as amniocentesis can lead prospective parents to suspend commitment to pregnancy, so the high-technology atmosphere of the intensive care nursery can lead some parents to suspend commitment to parenthood. As Anspach (1993) observed, the first experience of seeing their baby in an isolette, attached to a ventilator and hooked to monitors and intravenous lines, comes as a shock to many parents. This experience was so frightening to one mother that she reported having to put baby shoes on her bedstand every night to remind herself that she had a baby. In extreme instances, some parents become profoundly alienated from the nursery and withdraw from their babies. Such behaviors are viewed by some commentators and professionals as evidence of disruption of a biologically determined bond (e.g., Klaus and Kennel 1976). We suggest instead that suspending commitment to parenthood attests to the power of the social organization of high-technology medical settings to affect the emotional contours of a relationship that is consummately social.

Physicians, nurses, and parents, then, may all bring different levels of emotional engagement to decisions, levels of engagement that are shaped by institutional arrangements. But in the contests between these ways of knowing, it is detachment that is all too often asserted to be superior. As the previous examples show, however, neither mode of knowing alone is "correct" or "unbiased." Engagement can produce empathy, but it can result also in antipathy. Detachment can engender fairness or "objectivity," but it can lead also to objectification. It is only by bringing both engagement and detachment to the decision, by recognizing how each perspective can lead as well as mislead, that decision making can be improved. As Hochschild (1983:31) argued, "taking feelings into account and then correcting for them may be our best shot at objectivity."

EMOTIONS AND POWER RELATIONS

Professional Ethnopsychology

Discourse about emotions is bound up intimately with power relations. Close links exist among power, knowledge, and emotional discourse in the settings we studied. In the intensive care nursery, professional beliefs about emotions—their ethnopsychology—mirror broader cultural assumptions that emotions distort decision making, that dispassionate decision making is both possible and desirable, and that emotional distance improves the quality of decision making. In the nursery, this ideology is used politically to assert the authority of those deemed "rational" while discounting the views of "emotional" others. Some (male) residents, for example, argued that nurses were too emotional for their arguments to prevail: "I don't listen much to the nurses—they get too emotional. In every conference, all they say is, 'I don't like this baby, I like that baby.' If everyone made decisions that way, we'd all be in trouble."

Discourse on emotions figured prominently in early debates about who should decide the fate of critically ill newborns. Commenting on decisions about babies with spina bifida, Zachary (1978) argued that physicians should have the final authority in life-and-death decisions because the stress most parents were under would cloud their judgment. Although this argument is no longer used in today's nurseries, professional ethnopsychology continues to be used ideologically to limit the power of parents in life-and-death decisions. A frequently cited "folk" psychological idea is that parents who are asked to play an active role in life-and-death decisions would later experience guilt. We refer to this as ethnopsychology or a "folk" belief rather than a scientific fact because it has little support in the literature on the social psychology of decision making. Janis and Mann (1977), for example, argued that decisionmakers are more likely to regret the choices they have made when they are not given enough time or information to consider the alternatives carefully. In short, a well-intentioned but paternalistic effort to protect parents from experiencing guilt may, ironically, produce the very effect it is designed to minimize (for a detailed discussion of this issue, see Anspach 1989, 1993).

As is the case with neonatal intensive care, medical professionals in the genetic testing arena sometimes view parents as too emotional to make wise decisions, particularly when those decisions guide social policy, as the following example suggests:

> In April 1997 the National Institutes of Health convened a Consensus Development Panel to determine whether testing for genetic mutations that cause CF should be offered to pregnant women who do not have a family history of the disorder. When the president of the International Association of Cystic Fibrosis Adults learned of a conference at which major decisions on CF testing policy would be made, she asked the conference planner why organizations representing persons with CF and their families had not been invited. She was told, "We want the decisions to be based on scientific data. If we invite people who are not scientists, the discussion will be anecdotal or based on emotions" (for a detailed discussion of this case, see Beeson 1998).

Note how the conference planner alludes to a set of binary oppositions in which the "scientific data" of the experts are juxtaposed against the "emotions" and "anecdotes" of the nonscientific activists. In a single stroke, the conference planner draws a firm boundary between science and nonscience, between experts and activists, between reasoned discourse and emotions, and, in so doing, effectively excludes activists from the realm of social policy. This example demonstrates how discourse on emotions can be used politically to justify excluding certain stakeholders from critical decisions that affect their lives.

Disciplining the Emotions

So far, we have discussed how the discourse of emotions can be used politically to disempower and discredit. But in medical organizations, health professionals also attempt to control and discipline the emotional experience of their clientele more directly. One striking feature of the intensive care nursery's culture is the psychological surveillance of parents, that is, the extent to which professionals observe, record, evaluate, and interpret parents' behaviors and emotional displays (for a discussion of this issue, see Anspach 1993; Guillemin and Holmstrom 1986).

The preoccupation with parents' grief reactions and the nursery's potential to disrupt "bonding" has created a new role for nurses as emotion managers who monitor parents' behavior, attempt to foster "appropriate" attachment to infants by encouraging "bonding," and assist parents in "working through" their grief reactions. Nurses encourage mothers to visit frequently and to give breast milk. Nurses and social workers also believe in a version of the "better to have loved and lost" theory; that is, parents who "bond" with babies who subsequently die will have an easier time "working though" their grief. To this end, nurses encourage parents to hold their babies as the babies are disconnected from respirators while they are dying. Should parents be unable or unwilling to do this, nurses take a photograph of the baby, wrapped in a blanket, before the baby dies and present it to parents.

This psychological surveillance has far-reaching consequences for both parents and professionals who participate in life-and-death decisions. On the one hand, it diminishes the power of parents in decision making by transforming them from "rational decisionmakers" into "second-order" patients, as Guillemin and Holmstrom (1986) pointed out. At the same time, it empowers nurses and enhances their authority by transforming them into emotion managers and psychological experts.

Professionals in genetic testing intentionally or unwittingly manage the emotional responses of prospective parents by providing parents with certain kinds of information and withholding other kinds, as the following case illustrates:

> A pregnant woman who agreed to participate in a research project on CF testing was found to carry a mutation for the disease. But before receiving the CF carrier test results, she had been given an ultrasound examination and had learned she was carrying twins. She explained her reaction:
>
> > I was eighteen weeks, so they were already kicking. They were definitely there. Um, I'd already had an ultrasound, which for me made it tough because I'd already seen them. Something about that visual imagery of seeing those babies and seeing their little hands and their little feet and you know, it made it really real. And that, that was tough, too, in terms of thinking about terminating the pregnancy. That added a whole other element. And the fact that they were twins added a whole major element for me. Eighteen weeks pregnant was too late to find this out because you're already committed to the pregnancy, emotionally, physically, and everything else. I was really hooked into that because I had seen them and they seemed like little

babies to me. I had this whole identity in my mind—these two little girls, twin little girls.

The mother's emotional attachment to this pregnancy had been strengthened by viewing the ultrasound and learning that she was carrying twin girls, particularly because she had always dreamed of having twin daughters. After seeing the ultrasound, she became very excited about the prospect of having twins and optimistic that the twins would be healthy. Only weeks later were she and her husband to learn that both fetuses had CF.

Once the parents learned that the worst possible scenario had occurred, they felt they did not yet have sufficient information about CF to make a decision about whether to abort the twins. They contacted the Cystic Fibrosis Foundation and plied their physicians with questions. The parents' questions led to considerable discussion and disagreement among the professionals involved in the case as to what constituted "objective" information to be presented to the parents. The physicians agreed that the parents needed information, but they disagreed about whether the parents should be brought to a hospital ward in which children were dying of CF, an option that was ultimately rejected because of the objections of one physician.

This case illustrates the power of health professionals to shape both prospective parents' experience of pregnancy and their understandings of CF. Just as the mother's commitment to the pregnancy was strengthened by her experience of "seeing" the twins' "little hands and feet" on ultrasound—an image made visible by the instructions of her physician—so this commitment also could be weakened by the experience of seeing children dying from CF in a hospital ward. In their decisions about what information to emphasize and what to downplay, what experiences to reveal or to conceal, health professionals can have a profound effect upon prospective parents' hopes, dreams, and fears. Whatever professionals decide, their decisions will have a powerful emotional impact, and for this reason the goal of presenting only "objective" or "unbiased" information will continue to elude them.

An example from Lippman and Wilfond illustrates how written materials prepared by different medical specialists can elicit different emotional responses from those who read them. The authors found that information on CF and Down syndrome created by obstetricians for use before birth tends to be "largely negative, focusing on technical matters and describing the array of potential medical complications and physical limitations that may occur in children with the condition" (1992:936). This information differs dramatically from the more positive picture provided from the postbirth perspective in pediatric texts. In the latter situation, the focus is on compensating aspects of the condition and on the availability of medical and social resources. Lippman and Wilfond invite us to examine the educational materials we produce, not for accuracy—the facts are not in dispute—but to answer the more difficult question of why such different stories are told, whether this is desirable, and who should participate in writing these stories (1992:936–937).

In short, whether they recognize it—and frequently they do—experts who decide how medical stories are to be told or written are using their power to manage the emotions and shape the ultimate decisions of those who hear or read them.

Concluding Remarks: Emotions and Context

Our discussion of emotions in the moral life of medical settings has emphasized three major points. First, because most moral choices have an emotional subtext, many of what appear to be conflicts over ethical principles reflect deeper conflicts over emotional experiences and emotion rules. Second, emotions are not purely private matters, but rather they arise out of institutional arrangements. Finally, emotions reflect, sustain, and perpetuate power relations.

Over the past decade, philosophers and social scientists in many disciplines have become dissatisfied with the view of bioethics as applied ethics. To summarize what are more complicated arguments, the criticisms of applied ethics focus on three related issues. First, commentators have criticized the logic of applied ethics, the derivation of solutions from ethical principles. This deductive logic, it is argued, has little to do with how real people actually make decisions in everyday life (see Hoffmaster 1994). It is, to borrow Abraham Kaplan's fine phrase, a reconstructed logic rather than an actual logic-in-use (Kaplan 1964). Second, traditional bioethics has been criticized for providing an inadequate account of social action. Much of bioethics assumes moral choices are made by solitary individuals who wrestle with ethical dilemmas in splendid isolation from others. Actual moral choices, critics argue, are not merely matters of individual conscience but are complex, collective actions that are shaped by the social milieu (see Anspach 1993; Chambliss 1993, 1996; Fox and Swazey 1984). Finally, some commentators have criticized the politics implicit in traditional bioethics. The individualistic focus of much traditional ethics lends it a reformist quality that seeks solutions in disciplined reflection rather than in changes in the social milieu (see Anspach 1989, 1993). All three criticisms decry the absence of attention to a single missing element: context. They challenge us to produce better understanding of moral choice that brings context back in—both as an object of study and an object of change.

Emotions are, we suggest, an integral aspect of that context. Even when the various actors can agree on the principles at stake—and often they can—what divides them are the nature and quality of the emotional engagement they bring to a decision. An unattractive baby may inspire dread in a nurse and love in a parent. In fact, emotions often give principles their meaning. As we have noted, selective abortion for CF may feel different to a parent who has been guided to "see" her babies on ultrasound than to a parent who has observed dying children in a hospital ward. Physicians, nurses, and parents may all agree to the principle, "do no harm." But it is the emotional context that determines—as much as any other consideration—whether participants feel harm has been done in a particular case. As the plight of Roberta Zapata shows, "harm" appeared—or rather felt—different to neurosurgeons who measured benefits in terms of reduced blood flow than to nurses at the bedside who directly witnessed her suffering. A cut or a bruise, which professionals may see as a routine, small price to pay for ultimate health, may feel like harm to the parent attuned to the child's suffering. Emotions are prisms through which our principles are refracted.

Emotions are not only part of the decision-making context, but also, as this chapter has suggested, they in turn are shaped by other social contexts. To continue the previous examples, whether the various actors feel harm has been done depends also on a ward culture that separates doctors and patients, a medical hierarchy in which some give the orders and others carry them out, a teaching hospital that rewards its medical staff for research, and a society that relegates the task of caring for patients to low-status, female occupations, to say nothing of cultural views of children and disability.

Although emotions are central to those who make decisions, they largely have been ignored by those who write about them. In a sense, this volume is about bridging this gap between actors and analysts. Understanding how people feel about—and not just how they think about—the moral choices they make will be a small step in that direction.

NOTE

1. The alternative explanation is that these patterned differences between the responses of doctors and nurses result from the different sex-role socialization experiences of the members of both occupational groups, resulting in very different gendered moralities (see, e.g., Gilligan 1982). As Chambliss (1996) argued, it is difficult to resolve this issue definitively because of multicolinearity: That is, because nursing is a largely female occupation, it is difficult to separate the effects of gender from those of occupation, because both gender and occupational status are, in this case, very closely related. However, because most of the female residents responded similarly to the male residents, it is reasonable to conclude that the nurses' responses reflect their present experiences rather than their prior sex-role socialization.

REFERENCES

Anspach, Renee R. 1987. Prognostic Conflict in Life-and-Death Decisions: The Organization as an Ecology of Knowledge. *Journal of Health and Social Behavior* 28:215–231.

———. 1988. Notes on the Sociology of Medical Discourse: The Language of Case Presentation. *Journal of Health and Social Behavior* 29(4):357–375.

———. 1989. From Principles to Practice: Life-and-Death Decisions in the Intensive-Care Nursery. In *New Approaches to Human Reproduction: Social and Ethical Dimensions,* eds. Linda Whiteford and Marilyn L. Poland, 98–114. Boulder, CO: Westview.

———. 1993. *Deciding Who Lives: Fateful Choices in the Intensive-Care Nursery.* Berkeley: University of California Press.

Beeson, Diane. 1984. Technological Rhythms in Pregnancy: The Case of Perinatal Diagnosis by Amniocentesis. In *Cultural Perspectives on Biological Knowledge,* eds. Troy Duster and Karen Garrett, 145–181. Norwood, NJ: Ablex.

———. 1998. Emotions, Power and Policy: Structural Anecdotes in Genetic Testing. Paper presented at the 93rd Annual Meeting of the American Sociological Association, San Francisco.

Beeson, Diane, and Mitchell S. Golbus. 1979. Anxiety Engendered by Amniocentesis. *Birth Defects Original Article Series* XV(5C):191–197.

———. 1985. Decision Making: Whether or Not to Have Prenatal Diagnosis and Abortion for X-Linked Conditions. *American Journal of Medical Genetics* 20:107–114.

Bordo, Susan R. 1987. *The Flight to Objectivity: Essays on Cartesianism and Culture.* Albany: State University of New York Press.

Budetti, Peter P., Peggy McManus, Nancy Barrano, and Lu Ann Heinen. 1980. *The Cost-Effectiveness of Neonatal Intensive Care.* Washington, DC: U.S. Office of Technology Assessment.

Chambliss, Daniel F. 1993. Is Bioethics Irrelevant? (Review of Renee Anspach's *Deciding Who Lives*). *Contemporary Sociology* 22:649–652.

————. 1996. *Beyond Caring: Hospitals, Nurses, and the Social Organization of Ethics.* Chicago: University of Chicago Press.

Chodorow, Nancy. 1978. *The Reproduction of Mothering.* Berkeley: University of California Press.

Fox, Renee C., and Judith P. Swazey. 1984. *The Courage to Fail: A Social View of Organ Transplants and Dialysis.* Chicago: University of Chicago Press.

Gilligan, Carol. 1982. *In a Different Voice.* Cambridge, MA: Harvard University Press.

Gordon, Deborah R. 1995. Ethics and the Background, Ethics and the Body. Paper prepared for the "Humanizing Bioethics" research project. London, Ontario.

Guillemin, Jeanne, and Lynda Holmstrom. 1986. *Mixed Blessings.* New York: Oxford University Press.

Hochschild, Arlie. 1983. *The Managed Heart.* Berkeley: University of California Press.

Hoffmaster, Barry. 1994. The Forms and Limits of Medical Ethics. *Social Science and Medicine* 39:1155–1164.

Jaggar, Alison M. 1989. Love and Knowledge: Emotion in Feminist Epistemology. In *Gender/Body/Knowledge: Feminist Reconstructions of Being and Knowing,* eds. Alison M. Jaggar and Susan R. Bordo, 129–155. New Brunswick, NJ: Rutgers University Press.

Janis, Irving L., and Leon Mann. 1977. *Decision Making.* New York: Free Press.

Kaplan, Abraham. 1964. *The Conduct of Inquiry.* San Francisco: Chandler.

Keller, Evelyn Fox. 1984. *Gender and Science.* New Haven, CT: Yale University Press.

Klaus, Marshall H., and John H. Kennel, eds. 1976. *Maternal-Infant Bonding.* St. Louis, MO: Mosby.

Levin, Betty. 1989. Decision Making about the Care of Catastrophically Ill Newborns: The Use of Technological Criteria. In *New Approaches to Human Reproduction: Social and Ethical Dimensions,* eds. Linda Whiteford and Marilyn L. Poland, 84–97. Boulder, CO: Westview.

Lippman, Abby, and Benjamin S. Wilfond. 1992. Twice-Told Tales: Stories about Genetic Disorders. *American Journal of Human Genetics* 51:936–937.

Lock, Margaret. 1993. Cultivating the Body: Anthropology and Epistemologies of Bodily Practice and Knowledge. *Annual Review of Anthropology* 22:133–155.

Lutz, Catherine A. 1988. *Unnatural Emotions: Everyday Sentiments on a Micronesian Atoll and Their Challenge to Western Theory.* Chicago: University of Chicago Press.

Rothman, Barbara Katz. 1986. *The Tentative Pregnancy: Prenatal Diagnosis and the Future of Motherhood.* New York: Viking:

Scheff, Thomas J., and Suzanne M. Retzinger. 1991. *Emotions and Violence.* Lexington, MA: Lexington Books.

Scheper-Hughes, Nancy. 1992. Hungry Bodies, Medicine, and the State: Toward a Critical Psychological Anthropology. In *New Directions in Psychological Anthropology,* eds. T. Schwartz, G. M. White, and C. A. Lutz, 221–247. Cambridge: Cambridge University Press.

Stewart, Ann L. 1989. Outcome. In *The Baby under 1000g,* eds. David Harvey, Richard W. I. Cooke, and Gillian A. Levitt. London: Wright.

Weber, Max. 1946. Bureaucracy. In *From Max Weber: Essays in Sociology,* eds. Hans Gerth and C. Wright Mills, 196–266. London: Oxford University Press.

Williams, Bernard. 1973. Morality and the Emotions. In *Problems of the Self,* 207–229. Cambridge: Cambridge University Press.

Zachary, R. B. 1978. Ethical and Social Aspects of the Treatment of Spina Bifida. *Lancet* 2:274–276.

Zussman, Robert. 1992. *Intensive Care: Medical Ethics and the Medical Profession.* Chicago: University of Chicago Press.

Patricia A. Marshall

6   A Contextual Approach to Clinical Ethics Consultation

A lot of people say never give up. Others tell you to do . . . as best you can.
How do you learn to accept? Or do you fight "till the absolute end"?

Faith, a lung transplant patient

CLINICAL ETHICS consultation has become increasingly prevalent in biomedical settings in the last decade. A recent consensus statement (Fletcher and Siegler 1996:125) defined ethics consultation as "a
service provided by an individual consultant, team, or committee to
address the ethical issues involved in a specific clinical case." The primary goal of ethics consultation is to improve patient care by helping
patients, their families, and health care providers to identify, analyze,
and resolve ethical problems that occur in the course of medical treatment.[1] Central to achieving the objectives of ethics consultations are the
implementation of fair and accessible decision-making processes and
the improvement of institutional ethics policies.

The diverse professional backgrounds and skills of those involved in
ethics consultation contribute to the heterogeneous forms these services
assume (Baylis 1994; Fletcher, Quist, and Jonsen 1989; La Puma and Schiedermayer 1994; Ross et al. 1993). Despite such procedural variety, though,
the content of ethics consultations generally conforms to, and thus is constrained by, the traditional principles-based approach of Western moral
philosophy.[2] A philosophical orientation that emphasizes the justification of ethical decisions in terms of general rules and principles limits the
scope of the considerations that are deemed morally relevant and
ignores the emotional experiences and the lived realities of patients and
providers. It also extracts ethical problems from the broader social, cultural, and political forces that influence how those problems are defined
and understood, how they are evaluated, and how eventually they are
resolved (Hoffmaster 1990; Kleinman 1995; Marshall and Koenig 1996).
And although a principles-based approach does, by giving priority to the

principle of respect for autonomy, promote patient choice, it evinces little concern for exploring the meaning of autonomy and the impact of choices within patients' lives. Respecting patient autonomy often goes no further than eliciting superficial or simplistic answers to questions such as, "What does the patient want?" or "Does the patient have an advance directive or a living will?"

Invoking rules and principles in search of justification might lend moral decision making an appearance of objectivity. Patients and their families and the providers who serve them are not, however, the neutral, impartial, independent, and rational agents this approach requires. The individuals who participate in ethics consultations can be immersed in long relationships suffused by love and affection, resentment and enmity, or a complicated hybrid of conflicting feelings, and they can be buffeted by the emotions of sorrow, fear, and guilt that surround an impending death. Moreover, they bring with them assumptions about good and bad and right and wrong that are deeply entrenched in the cultural and social traditions that shape our understandings of illness and health and our beliefs about the use of medical technologies. For ethics consultation to be meaningful and responsible, it must confront those histories and those emotions and venture into the traditions and background assumptions that generate and frame ethical issues.

A contextual approach to ethics consultation follows this lead and situates ethical problems in the rich, complex experiences of patients, families, and health professionals and in the institutions and settings within which the parties in a consultation interact. During an ethics consultation, information about a patient's social background and significant relationships is gathered along with clinical data, but this information usually is considered anecdotal or peripheral. In a contextual approach, information about a patient's personal and social context becomes central to understanding the person upon whom the consultation focuses and to figuring out the reasons for and purposes of the consultation (Brody 1994a, 1994b; Hunter 1996). In this regard the "story" a patient tells can be invaluable. A contextual model thus reconfigures the form and content of ethics consultations by redefining and extending the boundaries of those consultations. And by engaging patients as individuals embedded in their physical and social worlds, an ethics consultant can be both an interpreter of and witness to a patient's suffering.

In this chapter, I use one of my own ethics consultations to illustrate the potential and the power of a contextual model. The consultation involved a woman who had to decide whether to pursue a third lung transplant.[3] A poem that the patient wrote in the course of making her decision, along with passages from her personal journal and notes from my interviews with her, allow her to tell her own story. My discussion has two principal aims: to emphasize how problematic and contested the notion of patient autonomy is, and to show how attention to context can change the nature and strengthen the substance of a consultation.

THE CONSULTATION

A social worker from the lung transplant team contacted our ethics consultation service[4] about a twenty-eight-year-old woman with cystic fibrosis who had undergone a lung transplant two years ago. She began experiencing problems with her new lung several months after she was discharged from the hospital, and she subsequently had a heart-lung transplant, following which she was able to return home. But a month later she had to be readmitted to the hospital. The heart–lung transplant also was unsuccessful. The lung transplant team rejected the possibility of a third lung transplant because it was considered to be medically futile. The patient was encouraged to consider a hospice program, and she was reassured that her medical problems would be treated and that palliative care would be provided when necessary.

Transplantations of a third lung in the same individual are rare. In this case, however, the conclusion that a third lung transplant would be futile was not unanimous. A physician who was joining the staff at another hospital to direct their new lung transplant center thought the patient might be able to survive a third lung transplant, and he communicated his opinion to the patient. If she agreed to be considered for a third lung transplant, the patient would have to move to the other hospital.

The patient faced a very painful decision. If she remained where she was, she knew that death would be imminent, that a potentially life-saving procedure would not be available to her. If she decided to pursue a third lung transplant, she would have to leave a hospital where the lung transplant team had become her "surrogate" family during the previous two years. The patient was given two weeks to make a final decision. During that time the physicians agreed to treat her medical problems aggressively and to provide her with supplemental nutrition through a central line—an intravenous tube placed in the chest—to encourage weight gain. In this way the lung transplant team felt they would be doing everything possible to reinforce her physical strength should she decide to try for a third lung transplant.

The staff requested an ethics consultation because they believed the patient was being pressured by family, friends, and hospital staff to decide one way or the other. The lung transplant team thought an ethics consultation would be helpful because it would give the patient an unbiased "outsider" with whom she could talk.

Over ten days, I met with the patient five times, and I spoke with the social worker and attending physician several times. I also met with eleven members of the transplant service to discuss their concerns about the patient's decision. At our second meeting, I asked the patient if she would allow me to tell her story in a book chapter I was writing, and she agreed (Marshall 1996). She chose the name "Faith" as a pseudonym, and she gave me written permission to copy parts of her journal entries for use in publications.

Our conversations lasted between one and two hours. At the time of our meetings, Faith was in the intensive care unit. She weighed approximately eighty-eight pounds and required a ventilator to help her breathe. Her dark brown eyes were large, accentuated by her thinness; her face was framed by long brown hair, pulled back with a band. Bright posters hung on the walls. Art supplies and several photo albums rested on the window ledge. Faith's journal was always on the bedside table. When I visited, Faith sat in a chair by the bed, with tubes connecting her to monitors and to clear plastic bags containing medications and nutritional supplements. The mobile tray placed in front of her always held water, juice, leftover food from breakfast or lunch, a pad of paper, and several pens.

This consult occurred because Faith was given an alternative—the possibility of another transplant suggested by a physician who disagreed with the team about her chances of survival, ostensibly because of his assessment of her physical condition. That option created a crisis for everyone. The team, out of respect for her autonomy, felt obligated to honor Faith's decision should she wish to consider a third lung transplant, particularly if that decision were genuinely her own and not the result of pressure.

Respect for autonomy dominates the traditional approach to ethical decision making in medicine, and its requirements seem relatively clear: Patients are asked about their preferences regarding medical interventions, and their voluntary, informed choices are honored by the medical team. In the complicated flux of clinical settings, however, respecting autonomy is considerably more problematic. Patients and their decisions are not patently and unequivocally autonomous; many parties participate in and influence the outcomes of decision-making processes; and decisions often evolve and appear rather than being formally and definitively made. Decisions, in other words, are contested, negotiated, and realized within the social and political dynamics that swirl around patients, families, and health care providers.

Attention to context evokes the social and cultural forces that simultaneously anchor and constrain an individual's freedom to decide and to act. It works with information commonly relegated to the background—shadowed and silent—and uses this information to recast moral problems.

THE PARTIES INVOLVED IN THE CONSULTATION

Family

In recent years, bioethicists (Blustein 1993; Hardwig 1990; Nelson 1992; Nelson and Nelson 1995) have argued that greater attention should be given to the family in moral decision making. Implicit in their arguments is the appreciation that medical decisions normally are made after consultation with family and friends. Faith's relational world was often contentious, however. Both of Faith's parents were alcoholics, and for a number of years she had no contact with them. Perhaps because of this estrangement, she became closer to her boyfriend's family.

The relationship between the two families was antagonistic and frequently resulted in emotionally upsetting interactions, particularly around the issue of a third lung transplant. Faith's parents and sister supported the decision of the lung transplant team, but her boyfriend, Joe, and his family wanted Faith to try another transplant. Faith wrote in her journal: "This morning [Joe's parents] came to visit early. I was really glad to see them. . . . Then [my sister] came and waited outside 'cause she doesn't get along with them. I hate that. I love them both. . . . They can't help but push a little." The difficulties between her family and Joe raised concerns among the staff. One day an argument took place in Faith's room. Her parents stood on one side of the bed, Joe on the other side; they were shouting at each other about who would be the beneficiaries of Faith's estate if she should die (Marshall 1996:221, n.4). The staff had to intervene.

Staff

Hospitals impose rigorous schedules dedicated to maintaining their administrative and institutional machinery—attending meetings, doing paperwork, making telephone calls, updating charts, ordering and reviewing medical tests, and so on—along with the surveillance and treatment of patients' diseases. In a journal entry Faith acknowledges the restrictions that the unit responsibilities of the nurses impose on their interactions with her: "The nurses are here but they can't come and sit by you when you are lonely. I've got to be able to occupy myself. . . . All these feelings are dying to get out: Anger, Frustration, Anxiety, Fear, Loneliness."

Faith considered all the providers on the lung transplant team to be part of her extended family. In two years of caring for her for months at a time, they also felt they had become very significant to her. Faith was aware of her dependency on the team and of her resistance to the authority and power the staff members had over her. She wrote in her journal: "I woke up in a horrible mood. Sick of being here in the same place, no patience for anything, being a whiner. All it does is make things harder. Jim is my nurse. I know I must piss him off. I got a big dose of Morphine and that just about knocked me out—so now I'm laying dizzy and paying for it. I bring this on myself I think." Faith's emotional reactions, her bad moods, have consequences, regardless of whether they are recognized as such by the physicians and nurses. In this instance, the consequence of "pissing off" her nurse is the morphine that knocks her out.

In her feminist critique of biomedicine, Sherwin (1992:92) argued that "patients are required to submit to medical authority and respond with gratitude for attention offered." Being a "good" patient means maintaining a cheerful disposition; complaints could result in hostility and impatience. Indeed, during several conversations, Faith expressed concern that the staff would be angry if she decided to try for a third transplant. Even though the staff repeatedly told Faith they would be satisfied with whatever decision she made, Faith was unable to dismiss her feelings of vulnerability and her fear of rejection—by the staff, her family, Joe's family—should she make the "wrong" decision.

The emotional vulnerability of patients is exacerbated by the dependency of being confined to a hospital bed. Faith is tied to her bed, metaphorically handcuffed to the bed, by the life-sustaining machines that breathe for her, medicate her, and provide a continuous record of her body's functioning. Alarms sound if something is not right, if her body begins to go out of control. Faith's emotions were certainly out of control as each day brought her closer to a point of reckoning.

Consultant

Faith did not request an ethics consult to help her make a decision. She understood that the transplant team requested my presence. She wrote in her journal: "I met with a woman from an ethics committee. . . . She's trying to help me make a decision from an outsider's point of view." "Outsider" is a misnomer, though. Although I was not a member of the health care team Faith encountered daily, I am a paid employee of the medical center and a faculty member in the department of medicine, and as a member of the ethics consult service for the hospital, I am, in my own way, a member of their team. Barnard (1992:15) observed that integrating ethicists into the clinical milieu may diminish what he calls "critical distance." That integration might also compromise the ability of ethicists to question seriously the values and assumptions of the institutions for which they work, along with those of the broader enterprise of biomedicine (Gordon 1988).

The Patient

Faith lived with cystic fibrosis her entire life, and she survived two transplants and innumerable hospitalizations. Her determination to survive is echoed in a journal entry: "I hope I have a future. I'm getting so scared now. I guess I'm not ready to die. Sometimes I think I am. I think of all I've gone through and all I won't be able to go through and all that seems inevitable and I figure it must be over, but I dream of so many things that I could have done. I want to laugh and be outside before I ever die. One more time. I want every second to count." A week later, Faith said, "I want to live without machines that breathe for me or one that pumps in calories for nutrition. Maybe that's asking too much. Maybe I already had my good time after the first transplant. But why am I still here? There has to be a reason and I have to figure it out."

An existential search for meaning shaped Faith's understanding of her plight. If she is "still here," does that suggest there is something more for her to do? Does it mean she is not ready to give up the struggle? Despite the portents of her circumstances—living with a body relinquishing itself to death, sleeping in a bed made heavy with the trappings of high technology tubes and monitors—Faith still imagines a future in a journal entry: "There are lots of things to do if I get better—drive a car . . . keep in touch with new friends I've made, clean my own house!"

But how Faith conceived her predicament is clearest in a poem she wrote.

> Riding on a bike, pushing with all your might,
> you can see the top of the hill
> so far away from sight
> push a little harder, just a bit more time
> if you can make the top, the ride down
> will be just fine
> you could stop right now
> put on your brakes, rest, or turn around and go
>   down easy; haven't you done your best?
> Listen to the people as they
> encourage you to try and push on . . .
> but your bike is starting to fall apart,
> the gears stripped,
> leaving you with the exact one you don't need.
> You hit a couple ruts and fall down hard,
> so hard you need help just to get back on.
> They fix the gears and tell you go on . . . keep going
> it's gonna get easier,
> something's wrong though cause you fall again, hard
> and this time the gears can't be fixed. . . .
> Every turn is harder now. Take a good look around you
> and look how far you've come.
> You did a good job. . . .
> A lot of people say never give up. Others tell
> you to do as . . . best as you can.
> How do you learn to accept?
> Or do you fight "till the absolute end"? (Marshall 1996:221–222, n.5)

Faith recognizes her own agency and capacity to act intentionally in her depiction of the alternatives and their outcomes: "If you can make the top, the ride down will be just fine, you could stop right now . . . or turn around and go down easy; haven't you done your best?" Although Faith is the one riding the bike, her relationships with others figure importantly in her struggle to decide what to do with the bike—with her "body." Faith acknowledges the support she receives to continue up the hill: "Listen to the people as they encourage you to try and push on. . . . It's gonna get easier." But her bicycle is broken, unfixable: "something's wrong . . . cause you fall again, hard, and this time the gears can't be fixed. . . ." Ultimately, Faith confronts her final decision, which she expresses, in part, as a conflict among her relationships with others: "A lot of people say never give up. Others tell you to do as . . . best you can. How do you learn to accept? Or do you fight 'till the absolute end'?" Faith uses the stripped gears of her bicycle as a metaphor for her deteriorating body. She has fallen hard several times; the gears cannot be fixed; and she knows she has done a "good job." Yet her indomitable spirit compels her to wonder whether she should "fight 'till the absolute end.'" Why is it so hard for her to "learn to accept"?

Faith's poem could be interpreted superficially as a passionate expression of her inner self and her considerable ambivalence about a third lung transplant. Her poem is, however, much richer.[5] It not only expresses the emotional undercurrents of Faith's experiences as a patient, it reveals the hidden assumptions that frame her dilemma. The metaphor of the bicycle is the key, for it symbolizes how deeply Faith has internalized the reductionist view of the person and the dualistic view of the relation between the self and the body that pervade our Western heritage. Faith envisages herself as dissociated from her body, which she portrays in starkly mechanistic terms: "your bike is starting to fall apart, the gears stripped, leaving you with the exact one you don't need. . . . They fix the gears and tell you [to] go on." A broken bicycle is taken to a mechanic to be repaired. A broken body is taken to a surgeon to be repaired, and, indeed, there is a surgeon who is ready and willing to work on Faith's body. The poem exposes how profoundly Faith's beliefs and values are structured by, and her judgment is guided by, the largely invisible contextual background incorporated into Western ideologies and thus into the ideology of biomedicine. Moreover, Faith has spent a considerable part of her life in a hospital, an institution devoted to a dualistic, mechanistic, reductionistic conception of persons and their problems. Her hospital experiences can only have reinforced the broader social and cultural mores imbued in her about the nature of persons, the relationship between self and body, and the promises of medical technology.

One week before the deadline to make her decision, Faith wrote in her journal: "I think I've only got about a week left before there's gonna be another meeting on what to do." The next day she wrote: "Lord, I ask for strength to get through each day and the knowledge to know what's right. I only want to do right." She records her decision three days later in the form of a prayer: "Dear Lord, I have faith in you that I'm doing the right things. . . . I'm going for another try for a transplant with Dr. Smith. . . . [Everyone—parents, sister, boyfriend—] wants me to go for it. They will all support me too, I can feel it. . . . Even the nurses here support me either way . . . I know Mary [nurse] doesn't think I'm strong enough but that's only opinions. You know the truth. I have faith that you will make something happen to lead me where to go, and so far it seems the signs all point for 'go ahead.' "

During one of our first meetings, Faith gestured to the monitors and tubes in her hospital room and asked rhetorically, "What is my choice? To live like this for the rest of my life? Or to try it again and see what happens? Is there a choice?"

DOING ETHICS

A customary principles-based approach to ethics consultation might focus on Faith's ambivalence and the pressure being exerted on her. Its primary concern would be whether her decision genuinely is autonomous, that is, informed, voluntary, and authentic or true to herself. And this ethics consultation was sought to insure that Faith was making an autonomous decision. But Faith's poem motivated me to ask a fundamental question in a contextual approach to ethics consultation: What does autonomy mean for Faith? If her deliberations proceed from deeply internalized social and cultural views about the nature of persons and the power of the biomedical paradigm, views that undoubtedly are magnified in the hospital setting that has become her home, what sense does it make to talk about her making an autonomous decision? Given the metaphorically revealing terms in which Faith poses her problem, how could she realistically decide otherwise? And if she could not, what should an ethics consultant be doing? Indeed, what is the point of an ethics consultation?

Brody (1994a:208) suggested that in listening to a patient's story one is likely to identify emotionally with the participants. But rather than viewing this identification as a "threat to objectivity," Brody believes that emotional empathy facilitates ethical insight by calling attention to morally critical factors. After spending more than a week talking with Faith, reading her diary with her,[6] and spending time on the unit, I developed an emotional attachment to Faith and the team. It was difficult to witness Faith's excruciating process of coming to terms with a decision that would mean either a remote possibility of an extended life or an imminent death. If I could have had my way, I would have wished for her a reckoning with the inevitable, an acceptance of death, and a peaceful reconciliation with all those she loved. I would have liked to have seen her accept the offer of the staff to arrange hospice care. I felt protective toward Faith and acutely aware of her vulnerability, my relative powerlessness, and her astounding will to live. I felt the enormous frustration of the staff, who cared deeply for Faith. I was outraged with the physician who had made what I thought was an outlandish and exploitive, if not coercive, offer of a third lung transplant to Faith; I believed he gave Faith this choice not because he really believed she might survive, but because of his interest in self-promotion. His action, in my opinion, was untenable. It placed everyone—Faith, her family and friends, and the team caring for her—in a terrible position. The team had been committed to Faith's treatment and recovery for several years; consequently, it was impossible for them to say now, "Sorry, you'll have to go elsewhere," without making an effort to accommodate her desire to try another transplant.

This situation could have arisen only in a clinical setting in which the biomedical resources, technology, and professional capability support the ideology—to a certain extent, even the mythology—that human bodies can live indefinitely. Perhaps my willingness to engage in extended discussions with Faith, to spend so much time with her, expressed my own need to reassure myself that I was acting in a morally responsible and compassionate way. Perhaps my involvement revealed my own desire to come to terms with the bizarre choices that biomedicine sometimes forces on patients and health professionals. I believe my emotional involvement did not hinder my capacity to be a witness to Faith's story and her struggle to decide, as much as I disagreed with the decision she made. In fact, my involvement caused me once again to question my own role in reinforcing the sometimes dehumanizing aspects of institutional biomedicine through my collaboration with the transplant team.

The hegemonic power structures within biomedicine maintain the traditional social order, in part by defining what constitutes a medical problem. The same phenomenon governs moral problems, for their identification and resolution depend on what is allowed to count as a moral problem. Faith's problem was formally defined as one of respecting patient autonomy, of helping her to make an agonizing choice. The need for a consult developed directly from the staff's desire to respect Faith's right and capacity to make informed choices about her treatment. Rather than conceal the surgeon's opinion about the possibility of another lung transplant, the staff were straightforward in acknowledging this alternative. Thus, respect for patient autonomy helped to create the crisis that resulted in the ethics consultation, and respect for patient autonomy was an obvious way in which to frame the reason for the consult—the staff said they wanted to insure that Faith was making an autonomous, informed decision about pursuing the chance of a third lung transplant. So created and so defined, the ethics consultation focused on patient autonomy.

In sharp contrast, there was comment about, but little ethical discussion of, the broader issue of a new lung transplant center at a competing medical center and the pressure on new centers to acquire patients for transplantation. The physician who held out the possibility of a third lung transplant to Faith probably was motivated by a number of factors, including the desire to "fill" patient beds at his new center. But the ethics consultation never reached the source of Faith's dilemma. As it was defined, Faith's ethical problem remained squarely within the borders of the intensive care unit where she resided and the borders of a conventional principles-based approach to ethics. Fundamental issues related to power and the responsible exercise of power, and to the missions of biomedicine and the subjugation of patients to those missions, were closeted. Yet those are precisely the issues that entrapped Faith, her family and friends, the health care professionals, and the ethics consultant. As long as they remain unacknowledged, isolated agonizing about the "autonomy" of Faith's decision is morally disingenuous. Perhaps such issues are ultimately too big or too sensitive for ethics consultations. If so, ethics consultants must recognize that although they might be able to do much to console and comfort individual patients, they can do little to initiate the kind of moral reform that would benefit patients generally.

In the end, Faith's decision to pursue the transplant was respected. For a principles-based approach in which respect for autonomy is overriding, the ethical solution appears straightforward: review the medical facts, assess the competence of the patient, determine that coercion is not a factor, and allow Faith to make up her own mind. In this circumscribed scenario, I, as an ethics consultant, became a facilitator of Faith's autonomous decision.

THE OUTCOME

Faith was transferred to the lung transplant center of another hospital. Her condition deteriorated, however, and when the day arrived on which she could have been placed on the list to receive a donated lung, she was too sick to be a candidate for transplantation. Faith died two days later.

CONCLUSION

Ethics consultation explores the deeply troubling moral complexities that arise in the course of medical treatment. The individual and social suffering that result from applications of biomedical technology create moments of crisis in which patients, families, and health care providers must confront decisions about what to do next. Sometimes this leads to the withdrawal of life support and reconciliation with the inevitability of death. Other times it means pushing forward with a panoply of aggressive interventions. In every case, though, these decisions are contested and negotiated within the cultural domain of biomedicine and the social worlds of individual patients and their providers. Inevitably, then, the ethics consultations that ensue are shaped not simply by philosophical assumptions about the nature of morality, but also by the histories and circumstances of all those involved and by the institutional forces of biomedicine.

Notes

Acknowledgments: I express my gratitude to all the members of the lung transplant team at Loyola University of Chicago for their frankness and candor in expressing their concerns about this case, and for their deep commitment to caring. In particular, I thank Dr. Edward Garrity, who discussed Faith's condition with me and was extremely helpful in identifying important background information concerning lung transplantation, and Nancy Jarecki, who spoke at length with me about Faith's story. I want to thank Faith for sharing her story with me and for the privilege of sharing it with others. It was an honor to spend time with Faith during the last few weeks of her life. Faith taught me about courage and persistence and vulnerability. She will not be forgotten. Finally, I am very grateful for the thoughtful insights and suggestions of Barry Hoffmaster. Our conversations about the case and the meaning of a contextual approach to ethics consultation contributed significantly to my analysis.

1. At the end of their book, La Puma and Schiedermayer (1994:203–225) included an annotated bibliography of ethics consultation and ethics committees and of the training and skills associated with ethics consultation.

2. This is, of course, an empirical claim, but one that has not been tested. However, in my experience and in my conversations with others involved in clinical ethics consultations, consultations generally are structured by and conform to the principles-based model set out in Beauchamp and Childress's classic text, *Principles of Biomedical Ethics* (1994). I am not suggesting that discussion of issues is limited to an explicit accounting of principles and their articulation in a particular case, but rather that a principles-based approach provides a familiar, foundational perspective from which to analyze ethical issues in clinical care.

3. In a previous exploration of this case (Marshall 1996), I was concerned with issues of gender and meaning in the context of decision making.

4. At Loyola University Medical Center in Maywood, Illinois, the ethics consultation service consists of three members (a philosopher, a physician, and a medical anthropologist) who rotate monthly on-call schedules for the hospital. The consultants are members also of the Hospital Ethics Committee; cases are reviewed retrospectively by the committee at quarterly meetings. Anyone may call a consult, including patients, family members, physicians, nurses, social workers, pastoral care counselors, and other hospital staff. When a consult is requested, the patient's attending physician is informed if he or she does not already know about it; this is done to reinforce our practice of working with the entire medical team on an ethics consultation.

5. I am grateful to Bruce Jennings for suggesting this interpretation of Faith's poem at a meeting of our Humanizing Bioethics research group.

6. Why did Faith allow me to read her poem? Why did she share parts of her journal with me? Is it because I am a woman, or an anthropologist, rather than a physician ethicist or a philosopher ethicist? I do not think so. Is it because I

asked to see her writing as a vehicle for establishing and developing a relationship with her? Perhaps. Would one of my colleagues—a physician ethicist or a philosopher ethicist—have used a similar approach? Possibly. But I believe Faith shared her personal writing with me precisely because of my emotional investment in her as a person facing a challenging decision.

REFERENCES

Barnard, David. 1992. Reflections of a Reluctant Clinical Ethicist: Ethics Consultation and the Collapse of Critical Distance. *Theoretical Medicine* 13:15–22.

Baylis, Françoise E., ed. 1994. *The Health Care Ethics Consultant.* Totowa, NJ: Humana.

Beauchamp, Tom L., and James F. Childress. 1994. *Principles of Biomedical Ethics,* 4th ed. New York: Oxford University Press.

Blustein, Jeffrey. 1993. The Family in Medical Decisionmaking. *Hasting Center Report* 23(3):6–13.

Brody, Howard. 1994a. The Four Principles and Narrative Ethics. In *Principles of Health Care Ethics,* ed. Raanan Gillon, 208–215. Chichester, U.K.: Wiley.

———. 1994b. "My Story Is Broken; Can You Help Me Fix It?" Medical Ethics and the Joint Construction of Narrative. *Literature and Medicine* 13:79–92.

Fletcher, John C., Norman Quist, and Albert R. Jonsen, eds. 1989. *Ethics Consultation in Health Care.* Ann Arbor, MI: Health Administration.

Fletcher, John C., and Mark Siegler. 1996. What Are the Goals of Ethics Consultation? A Consensus Statement. *Journal of Clinical Ethics* 7:122–126.

Gordon, Deborah R. 1988. Tenacious Assumptions in Western Medicine. In *Biomedicine Examined,* eds. Margaret Lock and Deborah R. Gordon, 19–57. Boston, MA: Kluwer Academic.

Hardwig, John. 1990. What About the Family? *Hastings Center Report* 10(2):5–10.

Hoffmaster, Barry. 1990. Morality and the Social Sciences. In *Social Science Perspectives on Medical Ethics,* ed. George Weisz, 241–260. Philadelphia: University of Pennsylvania Press.

Hunter, Kathryn Montgomery. 1996. Narrative, Literature, and the Clinical Exercise of Practical Reason. *Journal of Medicine and Philosophy* 21:303–320.

Kleinman, Arthur. 1995. Anthropology of Bioethics. In *Encyclopedia of Bioethics,* ed. Warren Reich, 1667–1674. New York: Macmillan.

La Puma, John, and David L. Schiedermayer. 1994. *Ethics Consultation: A Practical Guide.* Boston: Jones and Bartlett.

Marshall, Patricia A. 1996. Boundary Crossings: Gender and Power in Clinical Ethics Consultations. In *Gender and Health: An International Perspective,* eds. C. Sargent and C. Brettell 205–226. Upper Saddle River, NJ: Prentice Hall.

Marshall, Patricia A., and Barbara A. Koenig. 1996. Bioethics in Anthropology: Perspectives on Culture, Medicine, and Morality. In *Medical Anthropology: Contemporary Theory and Method,* 2nd ed., eds. C. Sargent and T. Johnson, 349–373. Westport, CT: Praeger.

Nelson, James Lindemann. 1992. Taking Families Seriously. *Hastings Center Report* 22(4):6–12.

Nelson, Hilde Lindemann, and James Lindemann Nelson. 1995. *The Patient in the Family: An Ethics of Medicine and Families*. New York: Routledge.

Ross, Judith W., J. W. Glaser, D. Rasinski-Gregory, J. M. Gibson, and C. Bayley. 1993. *Health Care Ethics Committees: The Next Generation*. Chicago: American Hospital.

Sherwin, Susan. 1992. *No Longer Patient: Feminist Ethics and Health Care*. Philadelphia: Temple University Press.

DIANE BEESON AND TERESA DOKSUM

7   Family Values and Resistance to Genetic Testing

THE PROLIFERATION OF GENETIC TESTING

WE ARE currently in the midst of a historic shift in the conceptualization of health and illness. Increasingly health and illness are being viewed through "the prism of heritability" (Duster 1990:2). The seductiveness of this perspective is reflected in the proliferation of terms such as "geneticization," "the genetic revolution" (Elmer-DeWitt 1994; Kitcher 1996), and "genomania" (Hubbard 1995:13). Lippman (1991:19) defined "geneticization" as "the process by which interventions employing genetic technologies are adopted to manage problems of health." She sees geneticization as displacing other narratives as it becomes the dominant approach to managing a whole host of disorders and disabilities. Regardless of what we call it, though, the essence of this historical shift is a growing tendency to view our bodies, families, and intimate relationships through the lens of genetics and to see our genes as fundamental to our future possibilities.

Although it is difficult to measure the extent to which geneticization threatens other discourses, it seems clear that biotechnology experts, government agencies, and health care providers have welcomed and supported the use of genetic testing. Carrier testing and prenatal diagnosis are desirable options from a biomedical perspective because they increase individuals' control over their reproductive lives (National Institutes of Health 1992:1161). Federal legislation promotes genetic testing of newborns. All fifty states and the District of Columbia screen newborns for at least one genetic disorder (Hiller et al. 1997:1281), and thirty-three states now have universal screening for sickle cell disease (SCD) (Lane 1994:157). Prenatal diagnosis and carrier testing have proliferated steadily since the 1970s. A policy statement approved by the National Research Council concluded that "couples in high-risk populations who are considering reproduction should be offered carrier screening before pregnancy if possible" (Andrews et al. 1994:6–7). This report affirms that "offering prenatal diagnosis is an appropriate standard of care in circumstances associated with increased risk of a detectable genetic disorder or birth defect" (Andrews et al. 1994:7–8).

Enthusiasm for genetic testing is not limited to experts. There is ample evidence of popular support for genetic testing. Attitudes, as measured in telephone surveys, are very favorable toward such testing, particularly among younger people and those who are better educated. About two-thirds of respondents to telephone surveys say they would want to undergo genetic testing themselves and that they believe the tests will do more good than harm (Singer 1991). A survey conducted for the March of Dimes Birth Defects Foundation by Louis Harris and Associates in 1992 found that 99 percent of Americans say "they would take genetic tests before having children to discover whether their future offspring would be likely to inherit a fatal genetic disease."

At the same time, genetic testing is not without its critics. Observers from a variety of disciplines (Asch 1989, 1993; Duster 1990; Hubbard 1990; Hubbard and Lewontin 1996; Lippman 1991; Rothman 1986; Saxton 1997) have raised cautionary notes. In recent years the strongest criticism of prenatal diagnosis has come not from religious groups, according to Wertz and Fletcher (1993:173), but from "some feminists and some advocates for people with disabilities" who argue that "cultural attitudes toward people with disabilities, directive counseling by physicians, and a technological imperative are implicitly coercing women to use prenatal diagnosis and to make painful decisions." Although conceding that "there are social pressures to use prenatal diagnosis in a 'technological culture,' just as there are pressures to give birth in hospitals," Wertz and Fletcher reject these concerns, asserting that nevertheless "most women, including most who consider themselves feminists, seem relieved to be able to make the choices implied in prenatal diagnosis" (1993:183).

In spite of apparently widespread favorable attitudes toward this new technology, a close look at the evidence for these attitudes reveals a paradox. The actual demand for genetic testing, as we will discuss below, has been significantly less than expected. This chapter examines this paradox by asking why genetic testing often is not used as extensively as providers of genetic services and many policymakers deem appropriate. Drawing on interviews with members of families in which there is an identified risk of genetic disease, we analyze narratives about family and genetic testing to understand more clearly the phenomenon of resistance to genetic testing.

WHY RESISTANCE?

We are not using the term resistance in the clinical sense of "noncompliance" because even advocates of testing view its nonutilization as legitimate. Rather we are using the term resistance in Foucault's (1990:92–102) political sense, to refer to elements of discourse that seem to conflict with or evade more dominant assumptions and priorities, in this case those of geneticization. We focus on the discourses some families employ in their reluctance or refusal to use genetic testing as a basis for making decisions about partner selection or pregnancy, particularly to elucidate the moral justifications contained therein. By examining families' moral justifications for rejecting testing and its implicit options, we hope to increase our understanding of how lay persons make decisions with strong moral dimensions and enhance our awareness of the narratives Lippman suggests are being threatened by geneticization. This is a particularly fruitful area to explore for several reasons: first, because the kind of research generally conducted tends to obscure nondominant values; second, because increased understanding of resistance may contribute to more accurate assessments of the social implications of the proliferation of genetic testing; and finally, because this understanding might also help to build a bioethics more sensitive to the deeply embedded values and commitments that structure our interactions with others and show how they are brought to bear on biomedical decisions. These three reasons are addressed in turn.

Resistance to new genetic technologies is poorly understood partly because most of what is known of lay perspectives comes from survey research. Although surveys efficiently generate quantitative data and in that respect have the aura of science, they tend to obscure nondominant perspectives. Quantitative surveys predetermine issues and severely restrict the range of possible responses, and they strip issues or questions from their contexts, thereby making it difficult for respondents to give realistic responses. Moreover, responses to surveys of the uninvolved public are based on very limited knowledge of any particular genetic condition and so are purely hypothetical. Yet survey research conducted in clinical settings inevitably oversamples those whose values are most consistent with a biomedical perspective. Relying on survey research consequently yields a poor understanding of why people resist geneticization. The alternative strategies of moving research to sites of local knowledge and reducing restrictions on the kind of discourse permitted on the part of the subjects during the research process are more hospitable to the uncovering and investigation of diverse perspectives about genetic testing.

Second, an understanding of resistance is crucial to the development of sound policies related to testing. From the earliest genetic testing programs to the most recent, problems and surprises have been common. The history of sickle cell testing is the best example of what can go wrong with genetic testing programs. These programs, initiated in the 1970s, often stigmatized individuals, facilitated racial discrimination, and engendered a wide range of administrative problems. Even today there is evidence of widespread resistance to sickle cell testing, including indications that test results often are ignored by those tested (Hill 1994a, 1994b). Advocates of genetic testing maintain that these problems are unique to sickle cell testing and reflect characteristics of the population tested; the problems encountered are not a more general rejection of genetic testing. They regard the experience with testing for Tay-Sachs disease, which was much more successful in generating community support and satisfaction, as a model and hope that it will be more typical of testing programs in general.

Other genetic testing programs, however, often have not had the high levels of participation anticipated in the planning stages. Levels of participation in testing programs for Huntington's disease have not even come close to early predictions based on surveys of those at risk (Kessler 1994; Quaid and Morris 1993). More recently, after the gene associated with cystic fibrosis (CF) was identified in 1989, commentators voiced concern that genetic counselors might be overwhelmed by the demand for carrier testing and prenatal diagnosis (Rennie 1994:94), but that demand has not materialized. A U.S. study reported by Tambor and colleagues (1994:632) found that "utilization of CF carrier testing in a non-pregnant population was low regardless of how the test was offered." Similarly, Clayton and coworkers (1996:622–623) reported, "We were most struck by how few people chose to be tested, particularly in light of the early predictions of widespread interest in CF carrier screening."

If we are formulating policies anticipating demand that does not materialize, we are wasting public and private resources. *Business Week Magazine,* in this regard, has described the genetic testing industry as "littered with corpses of start-ups" (Smith 1994). To formulate sound and prudent approaches to genetic testing, we must understand why and under what conditions expected demand fails to materialize.

Third, understanding resistance is important to building a bioethics that is grounded in the everyday experiences of those who actually encounter moral problems. For one thing, this approach serves as a safeguard against the danger Bosk (1992:159) alerts us to with respect not only to genetics, but also to biomedicine in general—allowing the technically possible to determine the substantively desirable. Nondominant lay perspectives, no less than the dominant perspective of biomedicine, are integral features of the social and cultural contexts in which ethical issues arise. Conducting empirical research that captures the full array of direct experiences of genetic disease protects us from the limitations of the abstract philosophical approach that has characterized much of traditional bioethics. As Hoffmaster (1991) has pointed out, one of the reasons ethical standards are in danger of lagging behind technological advances may be that ethical analysis does not pay sufficient attention to the lived experience of those who must wrestle with moral problems. Encounters with these problems must be viewed in social, cultural, and historical contexts. Hoffmaster challenges the simplicity of much ethical analysis when he notes that it is insufficient to regard persons as "disembodied rational agents with no particular histories or attachments" (1992:1). He points out that "this narrow, intellectualistic conception misses much of what constitutes the humanity of persons—their idiosyncratic pasts, their relationships to others, and their immersion in societies and cultures" (1992:1–2). Hoffmaster's critique accords with the work of Anspach (1993:35), who has described bioethics as "dominated by an image of an individual autonomous moral agent who reaches decisions apart from social constraints." As she effectively demonstrates in her analysis of decision making in intensive care nurseries, social factors are not "mere obstacles to moral choices, but the very stuff of which life-and-death decisions are actually made" (Anspach 1993:35).

In this chapter we explore some of the nonbiomedical stories told outside of medical settings by those who have a family history that includes a genetic disorder. Our purpose is to identify discourses that compete with those of biomedicine, not to deny the growing hegemony of biotechnology and the key role of genetics in that process, but to uncover tensions between it and other perspectives. In this way, we affirm the existence of coexisting and contending knowledge of human life and reproduction (Martin 1992) and the agency of human beings in constructing and choosing among alternatives. In doing so, we hope to increase our reflexivity as a society and thereby expand our potential to shape collectively our own future, goals that also should be congenial to a comprehensive vision of bioethics. We will discuss briefly our research design and methods before describing the forms of resistance we encountered in families known to have higher-than-average risk for a genetic disorder.

THE RESEARCH POPULATION: FAMILIES

This chapter focuses on resistance among families sometimes referred to as "high risk" by genetic services providers. These families are no different from any other families, except that at least one member has been diagnosed with a genetic disease or is known to be a "carrier" of such a condition. We report here on families in which a genetic mutation for one of two autosomal recessive diseases, CF or SCD, has been identified in at least one member. The recessive pattern of inheritance requires that both parents contribute mutated genes for their children to be affected, with a 25 percent risk of this outcome in each pregnancy. CF is the most common potentially lethal genetic disease among Americans of Northern European descent, as SCD is among those of African descent.

Although both diseases create chronic problems and early death is not unusual, life expectancy for both conditions has increased significantly in recent years. Only two decades ago life expectancy for SCD was estimated at about fourteen years (Diggs 1973:218). A recent study has shown that more than 50 percent of patients with sickle cell anemia (the most severe form of SCD)[1] survived beyond the fifth decade (Platt et al. 1994). Median survival age for CF has doubled in the last two decades to thirty-one years (Cystic Fibrosis Foundation 1998).

SCD affects the blood and is characterized by periodic crises in which clotting causes severe pain, organ damage, and possibly death. CF is primarily a disease of the lungs and the pancreas that tends to result in periodic hospitalization for respiratory and digestive problems and reduction of lung capacity over time. Both of these conditions are highly variable. Children who survive may be hospitalized frequently, but in many cases they can, with good care, attend school, participate in normal social activities, and even have successful careers.

Prenatal diagnosis for SCD has been available for over a decade, and carrier testing has existed for several decades. CF carrier testing and prenatal diagnosis are more recent possibilities and are significantly more expensive.[2] Nevertheless, both carrier testing and prenatal diagnosis are widely held to be the standard of care for both of these conditions in cases where a family has been diagnosed with the disease or a family member is known to be a carrier (American College of Obstetricians and Gynecologists 1992; National Institutes of Health 1987, 1990, 1997). Testing for CF is not routinely done to those with no known risk, but much consideration has been given to extending it to the general population (Brock 1990; DeBraekeleer and Melancon 1990; Rowley, Loader, and Kaplan 1998; Wilfond and Fost 1992; Williamson 1993).

THE RESEARCH PROCESS

The individuals and family members we interviewed were identified in a variety of ways, including in medical clinics and through advocacy organizations for individuals with genetic disease. We followed up virtually every lead we were given and traveled as much as two hours each way for face-to-face interviews, usually in the interviewee's home. When the distance was too great, we conducted interviews by telephone. When the affected family member was an adult, he or she was usually our first contact with the family; otherwise generally we began with the mother. Then using referrals we interviewed as many of the relatives as we could in a process known as "cascade" sampling.[3] Often family members referred us to other affected families.

We used a very loosely structured, open-ended interview guide designed to elicit narratives revealing the respondent's perspective on genetic disease, genetic testing, and related topics. Our goal was to limit the semantic structuring imposed by the interviewer to a minimum. Interviews generally began with the prompt, "Tell me about how you first heard about cystic fibrosis / sickle cell disease." Probing was used to clarify respondents' beliefs about the meaning of the disease for them and others, genetic testing, family communication on these topics, communication outside the family, and health care concerns.

We found that African Americans generally were much less enthusiastic about participating in the interviews and less willing to refer us to family members than were Whites. Payment of twenty dollars to respondents improved our success in getting interviews and referrals in both groups. Another strategy that helped us access African American families was to match interviewers and interviewees by ethnicity.

Interviews averaged about an hour and a quarter, with some as long as three hours. In general, the closer a respondent was to a person with SCD or CF, the longer the interview. The interviewers attempted to keep the exchange as informal and candid as possible. We did not ask direct questions about knowledge because it was apparent from the beginning that to do so created defensiveness on the part of the interviewee.

DESCRIPTION OF SAMPLE

We interviewed 180 men and women from 30 families with CF, and 189 individuals from 80 families with sickle cell trait or disease. Women in both groups were more willing and available to talk with us than were men, apparently because women are involved more directly as caretakers of affected family members. We had a higher level of participation by men from the CF families (38 percent) than from the SCD families (28 percent), and as the figures indicate we were able to move more deeply into the extended families of those with CF than with SCD. The two groups are roughly similar in that most of the respondents identified themselves as Christian, usually Protestant, with much smaller representation from Judaism, Islam, and various other religions. Both groups included about 20 percent who indicated "none" for religion.

The most immediately apparent difference between the two groups of respondents is that most of the CF interviewees reported their family income as $50,000 and above, our highest category, although most of our SCD respondents were in the lowest category ($10,000 and below). This sharp income discrepancy is not reflected in the education levels of our respondents, which are quite similar ("some college" is the modal category for both groups) in our sample. This pattern emerged early in our research and caused us to redouble our efforts to find middle-class families with SCD or trait. Our limited success in doing so may reflect patterns of institutionalized racism, but this sharp divergence also may indicate that SCD tends consistently to be more devastating economically to African American families than CF is to White families. CF typically requires at least as much care and usually more expensive equipment and medications. One possible explanation is that there is a much narrower margin of economic safety in SCD families. Women who bear children while young and single find it very difficult to maintain employment, and having few other economic resources, they often are unable to achieve or maintain a middle-class lifestyle. The SCD respondents were more likely to be single, divorced, separated, or widowed than the CF respondents. Their relative youth may have contributed to their lower economic status as well, because SCD respondents were somewhat younger than those in the CF group, with modal age categories of thirties and forties, respectively.

Prior to the advent of genetic testing, people learned they were carriers of these genes only if they produced an affected child, but among our respondents there were eighty-two (43 percent) from the SCD group and seven (4 percent) from the CF group who learned through genetic testing that they carried such a gene. This difference is not surprising given the newness of testing for CF and given that SCD testing is much more routinized in medical practice than testing for CF. California, where 83 percent of the interviewees live, has a state-run program (as do thirty-two other states) that tests all infants at birth for a number of defects, including SCD and sickle cell trait (Lane 1994; Shafer et al. 1996; Stern and Davis 1994).

PROCESS OF ANALYSIS

It would be inappropriate to make statistical generalizations based on the quantitative dimensions of our findings because random sampling was not possible or desirable given our goals. Our primary aims were to understand the range of concerns regarding genetic testing within each group and to compare the groups to illuminate general patterns and processes. In pursuing those ends, we identified key elements of social contexts that are linked to particular responses to genetic testing.

In analyzing data from our interviews and field notes, we were interested in discourse in its broadest sense—that is, talking, communication, and practices as they are revealed to us in interviews, observation, and informal conversation in homes, clinics, and other community settings. All interviewers tape-recorded interviews and supplemented them with field notes and case summaries. Working from both tapes and typed transcripts, we coded and catalogued all cases for both demographic information and characterizations of the respondents' perspectives on a wide range of issues.

We asked interviewees in both groups to sign consent forms identifying us as university-based researchers interested in issues related to health and genetic testing. In some cases people expressed concern that they might not be knowledgeable enough about biomedical issues to be helpful. Others often began by engaging in a somewhat biomedical and impersonal discourse, repeating what they had been taught in medical settings about genetics and genetic testing. Our probes encouraged them to go beyond this "official presentation of self" (Goffman 1973) and to reveal the experience of their private worlds. These personal accounts often are more emotionally charged and inconsistent with the front-stage public exchanges. It is from this interplay of front- and back-stage worlds that our current analysis emerges.

We draw heavily on the methodological perspective of grounded theory (Glaser and Strauss 1967). This approach is based on the premise that the best theory is developed from close engagement with the data. It involves an elaborate process of coding, or identifying, recurrent patterns, relationships, or processes found in the data, and the generation of conceptual categories and their properties from evidence using what Glaser and Strauss (1967:23) call the "constant comparative method." Negative cases, or cases that do not fit the emerging pattern, are particularly valuable in this process because they challenge the analyst to discover why this is so. This methodological perspective led us to a variation of "theoretical sampling," in that we made special efforts to find individuals and families to fill in missing categories. For example, early in our study we found many very poor SCD families, so we made a greater effort to find middle-class Black families. When we heard of CF families that had any form of genetic testing, we sought them out, and when interviewers traveled to other parts of the country, we encouraged them to interview families there. Usually, however, we took every available opportunity to interview those who fit our criteria because such cases were limited. Once introduced to a family member, we used cascade sampling to locate other relatives. But, to the extent possible, our emerging analysis was an interactive process with the data gathering. Our understanding of the central issues emerged from our engagement with the narratives of our respondents.

Our first concern was to clarify the processes that led individuals to genetic testing. We noticed that support for testing was part of the more "public" discourse with which our interviews often began. As interviewees went into more detail, became more comfortable with us, and began to talk in more personal terms, we found that the discourse changed—narratives emerged that were not integrated easily with the "public" discourse on genetic testing.

One common element of these narratives is that they were evident among respondents in all ethnic groups. Ethnic differences in narratives can be discerned as well and will be presented elsewhere, but we found these differences in many ways less striking than the tensions between the public discourses of genetic testing and the discourses used by the family members who are the subjects of this analysis. Members of both ethnic groups who utilized genetic testing usually did so as a result of initiatives on the part of their health care providers—a phenomenon Bekker and colleagues (1993) have identified as "provider push" as opposed to "patient pull." For example, we interviewed twenty parents of children with SCD who knew they were carriers of the trait prior to giving birth. Although fifteen of these women had prenatal diagnosis, no one in our SCD families had opted for selective abortion. In the CF sample, we found four children diagnosed before birth, but only one selective abortion for CF. It is in the narratives rather than in the numbers, though, that we can begin to discern some of the contextual sources of resistance to the geneticization of mate selection and reproduction.

FAMILY VALUES

The term "family values" has become politically charged because it is used to refer to a set of values that glorifies a stereotypical two-parent, religious, heterosexual family with children in which the mother is a full-time homemaker. Often the term "family values" is used to suggest that only certain types of families have coherent positive value systems—specifically those with hierarchical structures in which women are economically dependent and lack control over reproduction. It is this emphasis on structure that leads some analysts to interpret statistics on divorce, single-parent families, and abortion as revealing an absence of family values (Popenoe 1988). Arlene Skolnick (1991) argued that it is not possible to characterize the diverse sets of family cultures that coexist now with a single term. By following her suggestion and emphasizing value commitments in our analysis, we can clarify relevant dimensions of the social context of decision making regarding genetic testing. Here we are using the term "family values" to indicate that there are differing constellations of values held by families in contemporary American society; that these constellations are socially patterned; and that they often provide a frame that family members use to construct their responses to genetic testing. Later we will consider whether they bear some historical relationship to structural[4] dimensions of family life.

Our data reveal two broad categories of resistance to genetic testing. The first we call "culturally sanctioned resistance" because explicit narratives that have currency in the dominant culture support it. Within the broad category of culturally sanctioned resistance are two readily apparent sets of shared beliefs that reflect different priorities in family values. One is based on religious values, whereas the other emphasizes the values of romantic love. We label the second category of resistance "experiential resistance." It arises out of everyday experiences, habits, and practices but does not necessarily conform to explicit moral rules or principles. As a result, this form of resistance usually is more difficult for respondents to express or justify verbally, and perhaps for that reason their efforts at explanation tend to be emotionally charged.

Religious Family Values

Religious values are identified easily by references to God, predestination, afterlife, and so on. These values do not preclude testing per se, but often they are invoked to resist the use of testing as a precursor to selective abortion. Those with religious family values sometimes will use prenatal diagnosis to learn what fate awaits them, and perhaps as part of the process of selecting a mate; but with rare exceptions, they strongly oppose the use of prenatal diagnosis for the purpose of selective abortion.[5]

Religious moral justification also is used to resist prenatal diagnosis. For example, the father of two children with CF explained why he and his wife refused prenatal diagnosis with their second pregnancy:

We refused to do that. We didn't really care one way or the other, so we didn't need that, so we just [said], "Okay, fine, we'll just have the kids, whatever happens." . . . We said there's no sense because, [my wife] says, "Hey, I couldn't even abort the baby. If I knew, I couldn't abort the baby anyway," and, ah, with our beliefs and that, we just said, "Hey, that's not the way we want to do it. We want to have a child." Whatever it turns out to be is fine. . . . We're Christians, and we're fairly religious. . . . We believe that there is an almighty God that created everybody; and using that as a basis for our beliefs, we personally allow God to create whatever He creates. And so whatever happens as far as His creation, He has the master plan for everybody. He knows from day one until the end of it: You die and whatever happens that He is in full control of what happens and you're just, you're basically experiencing what life he wants you to experience here on earth. We have no guilt as far as something else caused and brought it in. If God had created these, this child, and decided that they were going to have CF or be physically disabled, whatever, that's His plan and His plan has a greater plan involved in that, and that is the growing of the people. . . . And we've had to grow a lot not only as parents, but we've had to grow with other people, interacting with other people through this . . . so that's the great plan.

Sometimes religious families are willing to go through prenatal diagnosis, but those who draw heavily on religious values usually make it clear that their purpose is not to prevent the birth of an affected child but to prepare themselves for whatever happens. As one young mother explained, "It is not up to us to control these matters, it is up to God." A young Mormon mother in her third pregnancy, when interviewed, recently had learned that her fetus was affected with CF. Her first child had died of the disease in infancy, but she would not consider abortion. She explained: "We believe that all this has to—in the end, everything we do on earth will help us to live when we die. We believe that we'll be together again, but a lot of people don't. They believe that death is the end."

The religious rationale for resistance to prenatal diagnosis or abortion or both is widely recognized and respected in clinical settings and has been noted in survey research (Singer 1991). The mother quoted above may voice what will become an increasingly common response; she justified the use of prenatal diagnosis on the grounds that because she lived in a rural area with few medical facilities, it allowed her to be better prepared to care for her child. This is not what most third-party payers would consider cost-effective use of prenatal diagnosis, however. Furthermore, there is some concern on the part of providers that accepting the risk of a miscarriage induced by prenatal diagnosis, although small, is unjustifiable in such cases.

Not all families or individuals who consider themselves religious reject or resist prenatal diagnosis. In one of our families, a Catholic aunt of a child with CF explained what she would do if she were faced with the birth of an affected child: "If it would have been early enough, I think I would have aborted. I don't think I wanted to bring a child into what my niece went through. I really don't. God forgive me for that, but I don't." At the same time she sees her niece's suffering and death as ordained by God: "That's just the way God planned it." She takes comfort in her niece's salvation after death: "And to me, Sara is blessed. At least she knew where she was going. We still don't know if we are going to heaven or hell. We don't know if we've been good enough to make it there. At least she is sitting with the angels."

Clearly she perceives a tension between her willingness to use selective abortion and her religious beliefs. Although her case illustrates that not all religious people oppose selective abortion, religious discourse is nevertheless a powerful source of resistance to using genetic testing to determine which pregnancies will be brought to term.

Romantic Love

Less well understood than resistance to prenatal diagnosis is resistance to carrier testing, which is often dismissed as a form of denial or irresponsibility by advocates of such testing. Nevertheless, this resistance is widespread, and often it arises from the belief that nothing practical, including carrier testing, should interfere with the quest for love. As Giddens (1992) explains, for "modern" family members the quest for love becomes central to answering the question, "How shall I live?"—a question made necessary by the disappearance of traditional work-family patterns. The break with tradition and the arranged marriages that often accompanied it has been facilitated by the emergence of the ideology of romantic love. According to this ideology, true love is not a response to economic or other practical exigencies. Rather, it arises from qualities intrinsic to the lovers. Rationality in the form of calculability, predictability, efficiency, and control—"instrumental rationality"—is inimical to the process of "falling in love." This ideology is expressed very clearly in the statements of many of our interviewees. If these individuals see a place for genetic testing, and they often do, it is not in determining who their mate will be. The selection of a mate seems to be one area of life where instrumental rationality is not regarded as appropriate.

Couples who "fall in love" may nevertheless use genetic testing as part of their reproductive planning and thus may face difficult decisions about whether to forgo having biological children (perhaps adopting instead) or to seek prenatal diagnosis and selective abortion to avoid genetic disorders. In vitro fertilization may become a viable third alternative, but this approach to reproduction was not evident in our sample. The modern perspective is that it is irrational to bring a severely disabled child into the world, but marrying for love is ennobling.

Carrier testing is more common among SCD families than CF families, but this difference does not necessarily mean African Americans are more likely to use the information testing provides as part of mate selection or reproductive planning. Often those who have been tested for sickle cell trait reject the relevance and implications of testing in choosing a partner, sometimes even forgetting their results or failing to communicate their carrier status to prospective mates. In many people's minds the term "genetic testing" means prenatal diagnosis, so carrier testing is not even considered.

One mother of an affected child told us that asking someone about his genes before telling him you love him would be "like breeding dogs." Another mother said that she thought it would be "kind of cold" if her children chose their partners "on the basis of trait instead of on the basis of love." Numerous members of both Black and White families declared that if they "truly loved someone," they would marry him or her in spite of the fact that they both might be carriers, and that "if it's real love, you can overcome things like that." One respondent explained, "it wouldn't make sense for people in love to break up because they are both carriers." Another discussed the issue with her best friend, and they agreed it is "better to be with your soulmate." In one of the few cases in which genetic testing became an issue prior to marriage, CF existed on both sides of the family. This couple made a point of refusing to be tested *prior* to their marriage, but they planned to do so afterward. Their behavior as well as their interviews indicated that they regarded genetic testing as permissible with respect to reproductive planning but not in the choice of a mate.

Thus far we have identified two sources of culturally sanctioned resistance, religion and romantic love. These two discourses are not mutually exclusive. Some people draw on only one; some draw on one more than the other; others invoke both. Although together they explain a significant portion of the resistance to genetic testing, these two discourses do not account for all of the resistance. In particular, they do not explain the decisions of high-risk, strongly prochoice family members to reject both prenatal diagnosis and selective abortion in spite of a direct threat of genetic disease.

Experiential Resistance

A third pattern of resistance to genetic testing is apparent among those who are, or in the past have been, particularly close to someone with a genetic condition. Because this type of resistance seems to emerge from direct personal experience, we call it "experiential resistance." In general, experiential resistance to genetic testing seems to reflect a moral commitment not to allow intimate relationships to be determined by genetic factors even when threats to health may result. Experiential resistance may be more apparent in deeds than words, reflecting embodied habits, perceptions, and values not easily verbalized.

An articulate thirty-seven-year-old woman whose younger sister died of CF when they were both teenagers explains her rejection of genetic testing as follows:

> We didn't know if there was a test for carriers. . . . It wasn't relevant for us. If any one of us were pregnant and it was clear that we were carrying a child with cystic fibrosis, we knew we would bring it to term. We wouldn't have wished that Janie not be born, and the thought of having a child because this child shared something that Janie had—it just created such cognitive dissonance in my mind that I don't even know what to make of it. I understand how someone without the experience of my family could think that children need to be perfect or else they're miserable, or we do a disservice in having them. But it has never been part of my expectation that people are perfect, or that perfect health means perfect happiness. I've just never equated goodness or life meaning with perfection.

The interviewer then asked, "What do you think about trying to prevent as much of this as possible through prenatal diagnosis and selective abortion?" She went on:

> It makes me sad. It makes me really sad. . . . Intellectually, I think a lot of people have kids and don't do such a good job, whether the kids are healthy or not. And I don't think we do a very good job as a community

supporting parents. As I said, parents of kids with special needs really need extra support. And that's the focus of my interest. I really rebel at the thought of fetuses being aborted because they are not perfect. There is something heinous and barbarous about that in my mind. And I don't feel a prejudice against a woman who might make that decision, but I do feel a certain level of contempt for a community that would try and support that kind of thinking, because it's so fascistic that it makes me sick. You know, I want to treat the people gently, but I want to be really hard on the issue, and I support an individual's decision to make that. But I'm really, really angry at a community that would try to encourage that kind of decision making or offer that decision in lieu of the proper support that a community should make available in raising a child.

At this point the interviewer interjected, "Are you suggesting that you think people might be making that decision because of a lack of community support?" She replied:

Maybe not consciously because of the lack of community support. I think they'd be making that decision because . . . my . . . recollection of the medical community's response to kids with disease, is that they don't consider them as human beings capable of having meaningful and wonderful lives that enrich. . . . It's not in me to make a decision about who lives. I don't think it is unnatural for people to be challenged emotionally or physically or mentally. What does seem unnatural is to try and engineer some subjective view of perfection. . . . I think disease prevention is fine. I think palliating symptoms is fine, but I'm against discrimination and I'm personally against abortion. I'm very, very much in support of a woman's decision to abort. I'm not at all in support of the medical community advising abortion on the basis of amniocentesis. I don't want to sound like I'm a proselytizing right-to-lifer. That's not where I come down on this at all. I understand that people would make those decisions. But I would want someone to make a decision knowing that there are alternatives available to them in the community for support, because I believe life has meaning.

Family members who resist genetic testing in the face of obvious risk may be difficult to understand, yet this response cannot be dismissed solely as an expression of ignorance. In one case, for example, a woman who was determined to avoid having an affected child had amniocentesis in her first pregnancy and again in her second. However, in the second pregnancy she was incorrectly told that the test results were negative. She and her husband sued the testing facility and won on the basis of a "wrongful life" claim. After living with this child for over ten years, she has changed her views and would not make the same choice again: "I figured I would terminate if . . . it's obvious that I'm gonna have a kid who has genetic problems. But, the actual course of [B's] life has been evident that that is not a valid stance. I mean her life is extremely worthwhile and valuable."

Similarly, the aunt of a child with CF drew on her experience with her nephew in discussing whether her children might seek prenatal diagnosis: "My feeling is that both of them, even if they knew they were pregnant with a child with cystic fibrosis, they would go ahead and have the child. They've certainly seen Joey grow up and function well with the disease. They realize he is just a normal kid. He's mentally healthy and he's physically able to do things. I would hope that they would go ahead and have the baby."

This affirmation of the value of life in spite of genetic disease is a recurrent theme among members of many families that have faced CF and SCD. Even when these conditions prove fatal, this perspective often is maintained. Janie's sister, quoted earlier, told us: "I think that the quality of life that she had, and that we had as a family was higher than the medical community at the time thought was possible. . . . I know whenever we talked about having fun and being basically well adjusted, there was just a little bit of incredulousness on the part of the doctors. . . . I just often heard my parents remarking that they felt the doctors didn't quite understand how it was possible for Janie to be living a normal life."

Although all people with genetic disorders do not feel the same way, many draw on their own experiences in rejecting genetic testing as a strategy for "prevention." A young man with SCD explained why he would be willing to have his partner have prenatal diagnosis: "Because then I will be prepared when it's born to deal with and know, and know what's wrong. Because my parents didn't know what was wrong with me until I was almost two years old." When asked about abortion, he said, "Umm, that's something I'd have to talk about with my mate, because, I mean, it depends on if I'm ready and if she's ready. But if not, then it may be the only solution." After he made it clear that he was open to the possibility of abortion in general, the interviewer asked him, "But what about selective abortion?" He replied: "Oh no! No, no! Because whether the child is sick or not, I'm gonna love him or her because I'm not the type of person who would disregard anybody because of they were sick or because—the only reason I would disassociate myself with a person is if they were a negative influence on me or if they just didn't respect me. I respect anybody who respects me."

In many cases, but much more frequently in the responses of African Americans, personal resistance to genetic testing explicitly is linked to the larger social implications of such practices. A mother of a child with SCD told us:

> You know, if I were confident that genetic testing would be used for the proper and righteous reasons, I probably would not have a problem with it. But I know that is not the case, and, therefore, I do have a problem with it. I know people will be discriminated against. I know that! We can say anything we want, but the facts are, have been, and will be that there will be discrimination. There will be unfair treatment of a lot of people as this becomes the rule of thumb or the order of the day, when it shouldn't be like that. I can see people even being divided up into groups. You know, you got all this, you can't do this—you know, dictating to people what they can and cannot do. And I think that is just wrong. I don't like it. I'm not comfortable with it because I don't think our society is mentally capable of handling it properly. . . . This is difficult because almost like yesterday, you could say you had a baby, it had a problem and you dealt with it. What is all this "you got to know what sex it is, you gotta know if it's going to be blond hair and blue eyes or brown eyes and curly hair?" People start picking and choosing their kids as if they are going to K-Mart. Come on! Something is wrong with this! This is real serious! I don't like it! We've been having babies since the beginning of time, but now they're made in tubes and we're picking and choosing. I'm not comfortable with this at all. Something doesn't sit right with this. I don't like it. I don't like it. I don't. Why do we need to test people? Why?

Experiential resistance, as we have shown, is found in families whose values emerged from, or have been reinforced by, their relationship with the family member who is "genetically imperfect." In the course of establishing an emotional bond with a loved one with CF or SCD, they come to appreciate the various dimensions of the affected person's existence, and the extent to which the quality of the affected person's life is a result of care and social support. This direct experience makes it difficult for them to assess the value of an affected person's existence in purely genetic terms. Family members become unwilling to equate the meaning of the life of a person with a genetic disorder to their disease, or even to the suffering that may accompany it. They are unable to avoid seeing many other fulfilling dimensions of the life of an affected person. Yet verbal articulation of these values tends to occur only when the family members are challenged by biomedical practices or discourse to act inconsistently with these values, and even then this resistance can be verbalized only with difficulty. This type of resistance is a result of direct experience with the genetic condition in question, but its verbal expression is impeded by the absence of an easily accessible, culturally approved vocabulary. The reluctance to apply genetic criteria to future offspring that is inherent in this experiential resistance seems to stem from a sense that to do so is to implicitly devalue the life of, and their relationship with, a living or deceased affected family member.

SOCIAL IMPLICATIONS

We have attempted to show that the processes of morally justifying resistance to genetic testing are strongly influenced by contextual features of family structure and culture. Although religiously motivated resistance leads to rejection of prenatal testing and selective abortion, and the ideology of romantic love inspires rejection of carrier testing in choosing a mate, experiential resistance rejects all forms of the "geneticization" Lippman (1991) has described as reducing differences between persons to their DNA codes. The birth of an affected child can be a transformative experience—a crisis in which families' values are reassessed and revised to accommodate new challenges—and families can come to reject not only genetic testing but also many of the modernist assumptions of control on which it is based. Thus experiential resistance seems to be a much more generalized resistance, not merely to specific forms and uses of genetic testing, but also to viewing intimate relationships through a "genetic prism" (Duster 1990).

Toulmin (1990:200–201) argued that movement into the "postmodern" phase of history "obliges us to reappropriate values from Renaissance humanism that were lost in the heyday of Modernity." He suggests that a humanized Modernity would no longer force us to decontextualize our problems within inappropriately narrow definitions of rationality that deny the importance of social conditions and social support to a high quality of life and to relationships with others. Toulmin's rejection of decontexualized rationality seems to be what the family members who are close to someone with CF or SCD are expressing when they resist genetic testing as a tool in determining either their partner or childbearing choices. They are seeking ways to strengthen rather than to sever social bonds.

Is it possible that the families who display experiential resistance are, following Toulmin's argument, harbingers of things to come? As genetic testing becomes available for characteristics that more of us have experienced directly, will there be more of what we have labeled experiential resistance? How will our existing family relationships be reconciled with genetic testing? Judith Stacey (1990) argued that there is indeed a new family form emerging, one in which the belief in an orderly progression of family history breaks down and family arrangements are increasingly diverse, fluid, and unresolved. She risks the hubris of calling it the "postmodern family" in spite of the fact that there is no one family type but rather dynamic household arrangements that reconstitute frequently in response to changing personal circumstances and that no longer reflect a belief in a logical progression of stages of family life. These families are postmodern also in the sense that they eschew the hierarchies and coldly calculating rationality that gained ascendance with the rise of science and technology. Our data suggest that values consistent with Stacey's concept of the postmodern family may be becoming increasingly apparent in response to advances in genetic testing.

IMPLICATIONS FOR CONTEXTUALIZING BIOETHICS

We have seen that members of "high-risk" families draw on a variety of discourses in addition to the discourse of biomedicine in defining who they are, what matters to them, and where they are going. This is not inconsistent with a hierarchical view of moral reasoning according to which ethical theories or the rules they generate are applied to the facts of concrete problems to yield practical solutions. But it does make the actual process somewhat more complex than it is often portrayed by reminding us that there are a variety of competing discourses available to persons who must grapple with moral problems. By using a qualitative, ethnographic approach that seeks the meanings that are central to respondents, rather than imposing preconceived categories on them, we have been able to uncover some of these alternative discourses.

The salience of these discourses in the lives of our respondents suggests that they may be as important in determining the fate of genetic technology as biomedical discourse or traditional philosophical understandings of the nature of morality. Because a coherent narrative of self helps one to negotiate the world effectively, more careful consideration of the various discourses people draw on could lead to more sensitive and effective social policies. Attention to the diverse discourses people use in forming their identities and in formulating action, combined with consideration of the potential for integrating these with the discourses of geneticization or other forms of biomedicine, would result in quite different policies than we have seen often in the past. For example, genetic counseling programs might spend less time focusing on getting counselees to be able to remember highly technical details and probabilities in favor of creating forums where people could examine their own values and prejudices.

The two "culturally sanctioned" discourses we have identified—religion and romantic love—link individuals with specific social institutions and practices. Although it would be possible to do an analysis that would distinguish varieties of religious discourse from each other and label them more precisely, more important, for our purposes, was the identification of other less well understood forms of resistance. After our interviewees reminded us again and again of the importance of romantic love as an organizing principle in people's lives, and we observed the difficulties they had in integrating this with the discourse of geneticization, it became clear that commonplace explanations of failures to utilize carrier testing are often too facile. What appears from a biomedical perspective to be ignorance or irresponsibility may, from another perspective, be an effort to embody a culturally sanctioned value.

One of our primary concerns in this volume is to contribute to building a bioethics that is grounded in the everyday experience of those who encounter new technologies. The concept of experiential resistance makes a particularly important contribution to contextualizing bioethics because it shows how technology is assigned meaning through local cultures and the microprocesses of everyday life. In the dialectical relationship with dominant discourses, lived experience is a mighty force. It incorporates the power of common habits and practices, shared commitments, emotions, and physical skills. As we have seen, this embodied knowledge may override both positive social orientations to genetic testing and religiously inspired negative orientations to genetic testing.

This qualitative approach to understanding resistance shows that although geneticization may be a continuation of old searches for perfectibility, management, and control over human life, it poses fundamental challenges to other deeply entrenched cultural discourses with deep historical roots. Virtually all of our respondents, regardless of whether they define themselves as religious and regardless of ethnic or biographical differences, made it clear they would welcome testing that is part of a process of caring and healing. As these narratives of resistance indicate, though, it is the strategies of calculation for the purpose of exclusion or destruction rather than the knowledge genetic testing produces that high-risk family members tend to resist. This attention to resistance not only illuminates the contextual pressures and supports for and against geneticization, it also suggests that there is more at stake in its proliferation than health and illness or the fate of individuals. It helps us to see ethical issues as part of a larger social fabric, because religious institutions, patterns of family formation, the meaning of parenthood, and the nature of the social bond are all implicated in the clash of discourses. The challenge for bioethics is to recognize and include these larger social processes in its analyses.

NOTES

Acknowledgments: This work was based on research supported by the Director, Office of Energy Research, Office of Health and Environmental Research of the United States Department of Energy under contract DE-FG03-92ER61393, entitled Pathways and Barriers to Genetic Testing and Screening, Troy Duster, Principal Investigator. The authors are indebted to Troy Duster, Robert Yamashita, Arona Ragins, Duana Fullwiley, Nadine Gartrell, Kristin Karlberg, Mark Casazza, David Minkus, Janice Tanagawa, Jackie Barnett, Christine Ogu, and other members of the Institute for the Study of Social Change who contributed to this research. We are grateful to the family members, their advocates, and health care providers who shared their perspectives with us in interviews. We thank Renee Anspach, Elaine Draper, Abby Lippman, Marsha Saxton, and David Wellman for helpful comments on an earlier draft, and the members of the Humanizing Bioethics research project for their valuable criticism and suggestions.

1. The term "sickle cell disease" includes sickle cell anemia, sickle cell–hemoglobin C disease, and the sickle cell–beta-thalassemias.

2. Beginning in 1985, prenatal diagnosis of CF has been possible through linkage analysis when DNA samples from both parents who already have a child with CF could be analyzed. DNA linkage analysis can also be used to identify carriers of the CF gene within the same families. Since 1989 this process has been simplified for the most common alleles, but linkage analysis is still necessary in some cases. See Wertz and colleagues, 1992.

3. Cascade sampling is similar to "cascade screening," which Williamson (1993) described as an effective method of screening. It involves beginning with known carriers and having them refer the researcher to biological relatives. Because we are more interested in social constructions than biological realities,

we occasionally included nonbiological relatives such as in-laws, fiancés, or fictive kin for their perceptions of family decision making and processes.

4. This use of the term "structural" refers to distinctive patterns of social interaction as well as to social organization.

5. One well-known example of this "religious" value system, not part of our study, is Dor Yeshorim, the program of the Jewish Orthodox Community in New York and Israel. This program originally was established to encourage carrier testing for Tay-Sachs disease and uses the results to determine whether certain matches for marriage are acceptable. They do this without disclosing the genotypes of carriers who are proposed as matches with noncarriers (Lefkowitz 1992). The severity and hopelessness of this disease were important factors in the development of this program, but now the community is expanding its genetic testing services so that they can be used to test for carriers of other less common and less severe diseases as well, as reported by Gina Kolata in the *New York Times* article, "Nightmare or the Dream of a New Era in Genetics?" 7 December 1993).

REFERENCES

American College of Obstetricians and Gynecologists. 1992. ACOG Committee Opinion No. 101, Current Status of Cystic Fibrosis Carrier Screening (Committee on Obstetrics: Maternal and Fetal Medicine, November 1991). *International Journal of Gynaecology and Obstetrics* 39:143–145.

Andrews, Lori B., Jane E. Fullarton, Neil A. Holtzman, and Arno G. Motulsky, eds. 1994. *Executive Summary, Assessing Genetic Risk: Implications for Health and Social Policy*. Washington, DC: National Academy.

Anspach, Renee R. 1993. *Deciding Who Lives: Fateful Choices in the Intensive-Care Nursery*. Berkeley: University of California Press.

Asch, Adrienne. 1989. Reproductive Technology and Disability. In *Reproductive Laws for the 1990s*, eds. Sherrill Cohen and Nadine Taub, 69–125. Clifton, NJ: Humana.

———. 1993. The Human Genome and Disability Rights: Thoughts for Researchers and Advocates. *Disability Studies Quarterly* 13:3–5.

Bekker, Hillary, Michael Modell, Gill Denniss, Anne Silver, Christopher Mathew, Martin Bobrow, and Theresa Marteau. 1993. Uptake of Cystic Fibrosis Testing in Primary Care: Supply Push or Demand Pull? *British Medical Journal* 306: 1584–1593.

Bosk, Charles L. 1992. *All God's Mistakes: Genetic Counseling in a Pediatric Hospital*. Chicago: University of Chicago Press.

Brock, D. 1990. Population Screening for Cystic Fibrosis. *American Journal of Human Genetics* 47:164–165.

Clayton, E. W., V. L. Hannig, J. P. Pfotenhauer, Robert A. Parker, Preston W. Campbell, III, and John A. Phillips, III. 1996. Lack of Interest by Nonpregnant Couples in Population-Based Cystic Fibrosis Carrier Screening. *American Journal of Human Genetics* 58:617–627.

Cystic Fibrosis Foundation. 1998. Patient Registry 1997 Annual Data Report. Bethesda, MD: Author.

DeBraekeleer, Marc, and Marcel J. Melancon. 1990. The Ethics of Cystic Fibrosis Carrier Screening: Where Do We Stand? *American Journal of Human Genetics* 47:581–582.

Diggs, L. M. 1973. Anatomic Lesions in Sickle Cell Disease. In *Sickle Cell Disease: Diagnosis, Management, Education and Research*, eds. Harold Abramson, John F. Bertles, and Doris L. Wethers, 189–229. St. Louis, MO: Mosby.

Duster, Troy. 1990. *Backdoor to Eugenics*. New York: Routledge.

Elmer-DeWitt, Philip. 1994. The Genetic Revolution. *Time* (Jan. 17):46–55.

Foucault, Michel. 1990. *The History of Sexuality, Volume I: An Introduction*. New York: Vintage Books.

Giddens, Anthony. 1992. *The Transformation of Intimacy: Sexuality, Love and Eroticism in Modern Societies*. Stanford, CA: Stanford University Press.

Glaser, Barney, and Anselm Strauss. 1967. *The Discovery of Grounded Theory*. Chicago: Aldine.

Goffman, Erving. 1973. *The Presentation of Self in Everyday Life*. Woodstock, NY: Overlook.

Hill, Shirley A. 1994a. Motherhood and the Obfuscation of Medical Knowledge: The Case of Sickle Cell Disease. *Gender & Society* 8:29–47.

———. 1994b. *Managing Sickle Cell Disease in Low-Income Families*. Philadelphia: Temple University Press.

Hiller, Elaine H., Gretchen Landenburger, and Marvin R. Natowicz. 1997. Public Participation in Medical Policy-Making and the Status of Consumer Autonomy: The Example of Newborn-Screening Programs in the United States. *American Journal of Public Health* 87:1280–1288.

Hoffmaster, Barry. 1991. The Theory and Practice of Applied Ethics. *Dialogue* 30: 213–234.

———. 1992 Humanizing Bioethics: From Abstract Principles to Lived Experience. Strategic Grant Application to the Social Sciences and Humanities Research Council of Canada.

Hubbard, Ruth. 1990. *The Politics of Women's Biology*. New Brunswick, NJ: Rutgers University Press.

———. 1995. *Profitable Promises: Essays on Women, Science and Health*. Monroe, ME: Common Courage.

Hubbard, Ruth, and R. C. Lewontin. 1996. Pitfalls of Genetic Testing. *New England Journal of Medicine* 334:1192–1194.

Kessler, Seymour. 1994. Predictive Testing for Huntington Disease: A Psychologist's View. *American Journal of Medical Genetics (Neuropsychiatric Genetics)* 54:161–166.

Kitcher, Philip. 1996. *The Lives to Come: The Genetic Revolution and Human Possibilities*. New York: Simon & Schuster.

Kupperman, Miriam, Elena Gates, and A. Eugene Washington. 1996. Racial-Ethnic Differences in Prenatal Diagnostic Test Use and Outcomes: Preferences, Socioeconomics, or Patient Knowledge? *Obstetrics and Gynecology* 87(5):675–682.

Lane, Peter A. 1994. Targeted vs. Universal Screening. In *Newborn Screening for Sickle Cell Disease: Issues and Implications* (Proceedings of conference held in Washington, DC, June 1993), eds. Karin Seastone Stern and Jessica G. Davis, 157–160. New York: Council of Regional Networks for Genetic Services, Cornell University Medical College.

Lefkowitz, Schmuel. 1992. Dor Yeshorim: A Grass Roots Success Story. *Genesis: The Newsletter of the Genetics Network of the Empire State* (New York State Department of Health) 4(2):1–2.

Lippman, Abby. 1991. Prenatal Genetic Testing and Screening: Constructing Needs and Reinforcing Inequities. *American Journal of Law and Medicine* 17:15–50.

Martin, Emily. 1992. *The Woman in the Body: A Cultural Analysis of Reproduction.* Boston: Beacon.

National Institutes of Health. 1987. NIH Consensus Development Conference Statement, Newborn Screening for Sickle Cell Disease and Other Hemoglobinopathies. *JAMA,* 258(9):1205–1209.

———. 1990. Statement from the NIH Workshop on Population Screening for Cystic Fibrosis Gene. *New England Journal of Medicine* 323:70–71.

———. 1992. Reproductive Genetic Testing: Impact on Women. *American Journal of Human Genetics* 51:1161–1163.

———. 1997. Genetic Testing for Cystic Fibrosis. *NIH Consensus Statement 1997* 15(4):1–37.

Platt, Orah S., Donald J. Brambilla, Wendell F. Rosse, P. F. Milner, O. Castro, M. H. Steinberg, and P. P. Klug. 1994. Mortality in Sickle Cell Disease: Life Expectancy and Risk Factors for Early Death. *New England Journal of Medicine* 330:1639–1644.

Popenoe, David. 1988. *Disturbing the Nest: Family Change and Decline in Modern Societies.* New York: Aldine de Gruyter.

Quaid, K. A., and M. Morris. 1993. Reluctance to Undergo Predictive Testing: The Case of Huntington Disease. *American Journal of Medical Genetics* 45:41–45.

Rennie, John. 1994. Grading the Gene Tests. *Scientific American* 270(June):88–97.

Rothman, Barbara K. 1986. *The Tentative Pregnancy: Prenatal Diagnosis and the Future of Motherhood.* New York: Viking.

Rowley, Peter T., Starlene Loader, and Robert M. Kaplan. 1998. Prenatal Screening for Cystic Fibrosis Carriers: An Economic Evaluation. *American Journal of Human Genetics* 63:1160–1174.

Saxton, Marsha. 1997. Disability Rights and Selective Abortion. In *Abortion Wars: A History of Struggle, 1950 to 2000,* ed. Rickie Solinger, 374–393. Berkeley: University of California Press.

Shafer, F. E., F. Lorey, G. C. Cunningham, C. Klumpp, E. Vichinsky, and B. Lubin. 1996. Newborn Screening for Sickle Cell Disease: 4 Years of Experience from California's Newborn Screening Program. *Journal of Pediatric Hematology and Oncology* 18:36–41.

Singer, Eleanor. 1991. Public Attitudes toward Genetic Testing. *Population Research and Policy Review* 10:235–255.

Skolnick, Arlene. 1991. *Embattled Paradise: The American Family in an Age of Uncertainty*. New York: Basic Books.

Smith, Geoffrey. 1994. The Gene-Testing Boom Is Still Set for Someday. *Business Week* (Nov. 21):102–106.

Stacey, Judith. 1990. *Brave New Families: Stories of Domestic Upheaval in Late Twentieth Century America*. New York: Basic Books.

Stern, Karin Seastone, and Jessica G. Davis, eds. 1994. *Newborn Screening for Sickle Cell Disease: Issues and Implications* (Proceedings of conference held in Washington, DC, June 1993). New York: Council of Regional Networks for Genetic Services, Cornell University Medical College.

Tambor, Ellen S., Barbara A. Bernhardt, Gary A. Chase, Ruth R. Faden, Gail Geller, Karen J. Hofman, and Neil A. Holtzman. 1994. Offering Cystic Fibrosis Carrier Screening to an HMO Population: Factors Associated with Utilization. *American Journal of Human Genetics* 55:626–637.

Toulmin, Stephen. 1990. *Cosmopolis: The Hidden Agenda of Modernity*. Chicago: University of Chicago Press.

Wertz, Dorothy C., and John C. Fletcher. 1993. A Critique of Some Feminist Challenges to Prenatal Diagnosis. *Journal of Women's Health* 2(2):173–188.

Wertz, Dorothy C., Sally R. Janes, Janet M. Rosenfield et al. 1992. Attitudes toward the Prenatal Diagnosis of Cystic Fibrosis: Factors in Decision Making among Affected Families. *American Journal of Human Genetics* 50:1077–1085.

Wilfond, Benjamin S., and Norman Fost. 1992. The Introduction of Cystic Fibrosis Carrier Screening into Clinical Practice: Policy Considerations. *Milbank Quarterly* 70:629–659.

Williamson, Robert. 1993. Universal Community Carrier Screening for Cystic Fibrosis? *Nature Genetics* 3:195- 201.

CATE MCBURNEY

8   Ethics Committees and Social Change

Plus ça Change?

ONE OF the most fertile sites for contextual analysis of health care ethics is located at its core—the operation of the institutional ethics committee (IEC). IECs have been contextual entities from their inception. They are the result of powerful social forces, and they represent both a response to social change and an attempt to foster further change.

In its 1983 report, *Deciding to Forego Life-Sustaining Treatment,* the President's Commission for the Study of Ethical Problems in Medicine and Biomedical and Behavioral Research recommends four roles for IECs: (a) confirming diagnosis and prognosis; (b) reviewing treatment decisions made by physicians, patients, or surrogates; (c) educating staff by providing forums for the discussion of ethical issues and methodological instruction in resolving ethical dilemmas; and (d) formulating institutional policies and guidelines regarding specific ethical issues. With respect to the educational mission of IECs, the commission stresses the importance of diverse committee membership and shared perspectives; exposing decision making to a range of contextual factors, from those that are case specific to those that are social; relating ethical principles to particular decisions; and having IECs "serve as a focus for community discussion and education" (President's Commission 1983:160–163). The promise of IECs lies in their ability to facilitate local, consensual decision making. The extent to which that promise has been realized is difficult to ascertain, however.

Most evaluations of IECs have not been empirically based.[1] Moreover, regardless of their methodology, these assessments have been concerned with developing or improving specific IEC programs, often on the basis of narrow internal criteria (e.g., outcomes), not with assessing whether the programs fulfill broader criteria such as those contained in the recommendations of the president's commission. A contextual analysis would examine the capacity of IECs to meet these expectations and would be cognizant of the settings within which

IECs operate, for example, the ways in which "ethical" dilemmas are defined, the processes that are established for resolving "ethical" dilemmas, the historical forces that impinge on IECs, and the structural constraints that inhibit the work of IECs, such as the hierarchical and gendered organization of health care institutions and IECs themselves.

An important study of Canadian IECs (Storch and Griener 1992) provides an excellent beginning for that kind of contextual analysis. Although this study did not incorporate the expectations of the president's commission, it exposed a serious impediment to the collegial decision making recommended by the commission—unequal access to IECs by health care professionals. The study found that differences in ease of access were particularly pronounced between physicians and nurses:

> Physicians seemed to have greater access to the ethics committees, and were perceived to have more support from these committees. In contrast, nurses were not perceived to have easy access to these committees. . . . The findings raise serious questions. . . . One overriding question is whether ethics committees support existing structures and power relationships in the hospital rather than provide a means for more collegial decision-making and increased interdisciplinary discussion of ethical issues and dilemmas. The comments from physicians, nurses and administrators give credence to the view that IECs merely support the existing power structures. . . . A second puzzling question is why the nurses might know so little about ethics committees. Is the lack of knowledge a function of medical politics . . . or a function of nursing administration maternalism which keeps staff nurses and head nurses removed from such information, or is it simply a problem in communication within the hospital? (Storch and Griener 1992:25)

These are troubling questions. Evaluating the policy and educational initiatives of IECs may reveal who participated in their creation and implementation and how effective they are, but that kind of evaluation is not likely to answer Storch and Griener's questions about who is not being invited to the ethics enterprise, whose voices are not being heard, and what the causes of these problems are. By excavating the social, political, economic, and cultural milieux within which IECs operate, contextual analysis can help find answers to these questions. And those answers could help to determine whether IECs are a genuine alternative to the judicial or governmental processes to which people traditionally turn when they are not being heard.

Access is crucial to the viability of IECs. Access for patients and families means knowing about the existence of IECs and their functions; being able to initiate and give consent for case review by IECs; participating in the meetings of IECs and consultations at the unit level; and receiving the reports and recommendations that IECs generate (Agich and Youngner 1991). Additionally, access for all parties, including staff, involves participating in educational activities or policy development, as well as contributing to the definition of what constitutes an ethical dilemma and the process by which it should be resolved. Needless to say, if staff do not have access to the ethics enterprise, it is highly unlikely that patients will.[2]

To address some of Storch and Griener's questions, this chapter presents key results of a contextual analysis of how one IEC operated. Although findings from this clinical setting are not necessarily generalizable, they do add credence to Storch and Griener's conclusion that IECs support existing power structures, and they suggest why and how that happens. This study found that an IEC's ability to resolve ethical problems collegially was thwarted significantly by impediments to access rooted in the IEC's authority and membership, the IEC's need for confidentiality, conflicting institutional work schedules, a tension between public and private personae, hierarchical relationships that created "insider"/"outsider" perceptions, and the more subtle influences of gender conflicts and competing epistemologies. In what follows, the setting and methods of the study are explained, the IEC's public or theoretical identity is described, and the aforementioned impediments to access are discussed in general and in relation to an illustrative case.

SETTING AND METHODS OF THE STUDY

Rest Haven, a Roman Catholic long-term care center located in a Canadian city, was the setting for this research project.[3] The facility, which is owned and operated by a women's religious community, combines a home for the aged and a hospital for persons with chronic conditions. This site was chosen in part because the facility acquired an ethicist and established its IEC in 1981, earlier than most Canadian facilities, especially those providing long-term care. It was thought that the longevity and multidimensional nature of this ethics enterprise could provide the basis for a robust contextual analysis, for it could be investigated not only in relation to factors influencing the growth and development of IECs generally, but also in relation to factors pertinent to this IEC's Catholic roots and ongoing Catholic ethos. The research began in 1991, the IEC's tenth-anniversary year, and was completed in 1993.

The methodology was primarily ethnographic, that is, an attempt to provide " 'thick' or dense descriptions of ongoing social processes and insight into the meaning of actions and events from participants' points of view" (Kelly et al. 1997:137). To describe the ongoing social life of the Rest Haven IEC, I collected data through participant observation, review of pertinent documents, and interviews. During the 1991–1992 committee year at Rest Haven, I attended all IEC meetings as an observer, and I participated occasionally when I was asked to contribute to discussions. I also studied minutes of all the IEC's meetings, all documents the IEC produced, all correspondence that the committee initiated and to which it responded, and pertinent structural documents, for example, the IEC's terms of reference, Rest Haven's organizational charts, and relevant archival material. In addition, I conducted audiotaped face-to-face interviews (two or three one-hour interviews per person) with most of the IEC's 1991–1992 membership (i.e., eleven out of seventeen members including the ethicists), and six members of the IEC's pre-1991 memberships whose collective tenure spanned the entire life of the IEC. Six of the IEC's eleven original members were interviewed, four of whom served on the IEC for eight or more years. The 1991–1992 membership included four physicians, five administrators, two ethicists, one nurse team leader, one resident of the Home for the Aged, and one representative each from the Pastoral Care, Education, and Social Work Departments and from Palliative Care.

The methodology also included elements not necessarily part of ethnographies, for example, an analysis of the history of the Rest Haven IEC (e.g., key turning points, major developmental stages, influence of important events), a study of structural factors (e.g., economic, political, social, cultural), an investigation of key values operative in the life of the Rest Haven IEC (e.g., individualism/community, competition/cooperation, equality/hierarchy, pragmatism/prophecy), and a review of indicators of the future direction of ethics at Rest Haven (Holland and Henriot 1989:98–101; see also Mount 1990). The history was developed on the basis of the IEC's minutes, veteran members' recollections, and one view of the developmental stages of IECs (Allatt and Sheehan 1992).

Major structural considerations included the overall organization of the facility, the effect of governmental directives regarding alterations to the delivery of long-term care, and the influence of Roman Catholicism.

ACCESS TO THE REST HAVEN IEC

In 1981, the Sister Administrator of Rest Haven communicated with diocesan Catholic officials to begin the process of establishing an IEC in the facility. The sister's wish to create an IEC derived from many factors, including the absence of facility guidelines for dealing with ethical dilemmas related to resuscitation, physicians' recognition that clinical decision making increasingly involved a more educated public and quality-of-life issues, and a call for the establishment of IECs from North American bishops' conferences and Catholic health associations. Diocesan officials appointed a priest moral theologian to guide the Rest Haven IEC, and by 1982 a lay theologian ethicist was hired to serve Rest Haven and the other health care facilities owned by these sisters.

As a standing committee of the board of directors from its inception, the Rest Haven IEC attempted to fulfill two of the four roles suggested by the president's commission: educating staff and formulating institutional policies on ethical issues. Ethical guidance regarding specific treatment decisions was provided by the theologian ethicists at the unit level, so the IEC itself was not involved in individual cases except when an accumulation of certain categories of cases precipitated policy development.

In 1987, Rest Haven issued a policy to facilitate access to the IEC and the ethicists. The policy stated that "all physicians, staff multidisciplinary care teams, institutional committees, volunteers, patients, residents and their families" had access to the IEC. By this point, Ethics Consultant had become the ethicists' title, and the access policy provided that "the Ethics Consultant is also available to individuals/groups for discussion of individual cases." The procedure for gaining access to the IEC, which follows, did not indicate what criteria would be used to decide which issues were "appropriate" for discussion by the IEC:

1. Any individual of the multidisciplinary care team and/or committee may ask the Ethics Committee to consider an issue.
2. A meeting will be arranged with the initiator of the request, the chairperson of the Ethics Committee (Medical Director) and the Ethics Consultant. The agenda of this meeting is to determine: (a) whether

the issue is appropriate to be addressed by the Ethics Committee; (b) the best approach for presenting the issue to the Committee; (c) what information is required; (d) who has an interest and viewpoint on the particular issue and how these persons will be invited to participate in the meeting.

3. The issue will be placed on the Ethics Committee Agenda at the discretion of the Chairperson.

Virtually all of the 1991–1992 IEC members told me that although this policy in principle provided for open access to the Ethics Consultant and the IEC via an initial exploratory meeting, access was in practice significantly limited, for a variety of reasons.

Access was impeded because IEC members were confused about whether they represented themselves or a given constituency. Fears about elitism are reflected in one member's comments about privileged access to written information: "The committee members [get information]. But why do the committee members get it? Do they get it just to have a full box of information that nobody else has? Do we get it to inform our own departments or programs—to make sure that other people have access to it?" The same member spoke about the tension between the confidentiality required by the IEC and the IEC's public emphasis on facilitywide communication:

> I always get the sense that when we do something on the ethics committee, it is confidential and we can't publicize it until we come to a decision; but then decisions are three or four months down the road or we never get there. So how do you communicate? If you do tell people where we're going to go at the next committee meeting, they ask questions and then other people get upset because questions are asked. I think lack of communication, communication skills, and a basic process of communicating down the line to the grassroots is not only the problem of the ethics committee, but of this whole facility and any large facility. . . . I think the more that people give little information, the more the grapevine goes to work and fills in missing pieces.

The problems generated by lack of input from front-line staff because of the perceived requirements of confidentiality, and by the ensuing misinformation spread through the grapevine, were aggravated by conflicting work schedules. Although few of the front-line staff rotated shifts and some constantly worked evenings or nights, the work of the IEC and the ethicists generally was restricted to the day shift. The staff's access to the educational opportunities provided by the Ethics Consultant and the IEC, and to the help that education might give them, was consequently restricted. Nurses particularly were affected, as one IEC member recalls:

> I never get a sense from within departments or programs or units that people are encouraged to go [to the Ethics Rounds]. I think the sense is that the people who go must have a very easy job because they have the freedom to take the time off. . . . Now granted, my time is flexible—more flexible than that of a nurse. How do you get this [education] down to nurses on the units? Within our program . . . how we chose to handle it was to have [Ethicist X] come in to take one of our multidisciplinary meetings. . . . It was excellent and it was great for those who were there. But who wasn't there? The nurses on the floor. . . . Who's shortchanged? It's the grassroots people who get shortchanged. Who has to make decisions in a hurry? The grassroots people. Who do the families ask questions of from 3:30 until 7:30 in the morning? The nurses! They're never here for the in-services. . . . Is this what's supposed to happen? . . . What access do they have to education in order to make a big decision? How much emphasis does the facility put on helping them to make a big decision? I think they're the forgotten ones.

At Rest Haven, many people said that the IEC's lofty position as a board committee was indicative of the vital importance of ethics within the organization and of the IEC's and the ethicists' facilitywide mandate. But the administrative status of the IEC thwarted access in two important respects: Administrative concerns about control sometimes stifled ethical reflection, and the almost exclusively middle-manager membership created a gap between the bedside and the committee. One member explained the former in these words: "The ethics committee is at the top of the pyramid. Hence, there's the appearance of a critique, but it's muffled. On one side of the coin, this [placement] is a way of communicating how important ethics is; but it's also a way of keeping ethics close to the security of top management control. The members of the ethics committee are blinded by being at the top."

The gap between the IEC and the bedside was detrimental to both IEC members and front-line staff. For the members, this gap hampered awareness of bedside ethical concerns:

> It's really the bedside caregiver who expresses the concerns; but this is not a caregiver committee. That causes ambivalence and we—I don't know what goes on at the bedside. . . . We can say that these are the kinds of things we want to do; but then when it gets transmitted down to patients

and it involves families whom you don't know and who don't know where you're coming from . . . it becomes very difficult! There's a great gap between the delivery of service, if you will, and the people who are sitting on that committee.

IEC members were not only hierarchically removed from the staff at the bedside, they were also, as one person suggests, distanced from "outsiders"—the evening and night front-line staff who, although ineligible for IEC membership, nevertheless found themselves subject to the IEC's daytime-based authority:

The evening and night staff—who are sometimes seen as outsiders—are complaining that rules are created and imposed by daytimers, but that they are the ones who have to carry them out. The ethics committee—its membership—has been confronted by this in terms of questions being raised about membership—having front-line caregivers on the committee. There were forces that said, "No, they're not smart enough; no, they're not high enough; no, they're not strong enough; no, they're too busy . . . they're chained to the bedside; they're foreign to us; they don't belong to us."

The contrast between the IEC's public projection of open access and the more private reality of limited access was paralleled by the tension IEC members experienced between their public personae as expert professional caregivers and their personal vulnerabilities and struggles with ethical issues. As one member commented, this tension contributed to a reluctance to have a patient or resident on the committee: "God forbid that we should have a patient or resident on the committee. We don't want to talk in front of them because then they'll know how we really are. This is an elusive reality. You don't see it named in the minutes really, but it's there. If you read between the lines, you can see it. . . . There are structural barriers that are so insidious, and they have a life of their own and they force people into boxes and into channels that they ought not to be in if we are truly focused on who the patients and residents are."

During the 1991–1992 year, a resident joined the IEC for the first time in the committee's history. When I asked a veteran member why this took so long to occur, I was given this answer:

We didn't have a resident before because we wanted to be free to discuss things more openly. There was a feeling that having a resident there would inhibit our discussion. It [i.e., the current membership] represents the concern that . . . we may not be reaching people directly. I think we were partly insecure; we wanted to be able to discuss things that were dilemmas for us and to reach our solutions together without having a patient or resident there, i.e., so that we could look at how we felt without having. . . . I think we intentionally did not have a patient or resident there.

Recognizing these types of impediments to access, many have argued that a lone ethics consultant or a consultation team composed of two or three people would be more mobile and better positioned at the local level to engage front-line staff, patients, and families in genuine consensual dialogue. My research indicates, however, that this model of case consultation encounters the same obstacles to access as consultation by committee. When I asked an IEC member whether front-line staff, for instance, a staff nurse, could initiate a consultation, I was told: "Nurses usually have gone through the unit administrator (UA) and the director of nursing. It really was quite threatening for a staff person to approach the committee personally. . . . I don't think that it has ever worked that they are able to initiate a consultation. It has always come through the hierarchy. We've said that a nurse can call an ethicist, but I don't think she'd dare. Ask the ethicists if it has ever happened. I would think not. I think the hierarchy is just too strongly established."

One of the ethicists verified this impression:

Yes, it's almost always—it would be unit administrators (UAs) and/or physicians [who call me] and when it has been people other than that— well, like staff social workers have called me up and organized a consultation. But it's almost always been the attending physician or the UA who has arranged the meeting. That's what has happened in terms of access. Individuals have accessed us and spoken to us one-on-one about concerns that they have, and if an individual phones and speaks with me about wanting to talk about a problem on the floor, they're welcome to do that. . . . What I do is ask them to speak to a physician and to the UA and say that they would like to have some discussion about this question. The physician or the UA, for example, might say that the problem in question is none of their business, and that they are not going to call an ethics meeting about a patient-care policy.

Other people have come individually and expressed their concerns, and when I have encouraged them to communicate those concerns, they have either said, "I have to work with these people every day and I don't want to take it further," or, "I'm not prepared to do that and I'd rather leave than do that." How far people pursue their concerns is a mystery to me, and that's where I see the possibility of my perpetuating a hierarchical relationship [e.g., between physicians and nurses]. It's fine to say that everyone has access to me; but if in reality that only works when key players agree to that—to the issue being discussed seriously—what does access mean?

The ethicist's description of the situation confirms that, in practice, access to consultation requires an endorsement from those who hold authority and power in health care and thus is contingent upon the practical implications of challenging that hierarchy. The ethicist's words illustrate and support Storch and Griener's hypothesis that physicians and UAs act as "gatekeepers" to consultation. The ethicist's answer also emphasizes that there is a substantial difference between access to the ethicist's understanding ear and access to consensual, interdisciplinary discussions of ethical issues. Consequently, "access" for someone lower in the institutional hierarchy may simply preserve the status quo, as the following vignette illustrates.

IMPEDIMENTS TO ACCESS: AN ILLUSTRATIVE CASE

Although a group of nurses achieved access to one of the ethicists and the Rest Haven IEC, the underlying social structures prevented consensual, interdisciplinary discussion of their concerns. Indeed, genuine ethical differences between the nurses and the others involved were minimized if not obliterated. This deflation occurred as a result of disregard for or delegitimization of the nurses' stand on the issues—a dismissal that had hierarchical, gender, and epistemological underpinnings. The troubling situation involved a dying patient whose family had decided, in consultation with the attending physician, that no artificial nutrition or hydration would be provided. The ethicist's and the IEC's review of the situation ultimately was retrospective because the patient died just before the ethicist's first meeting with the family and the nursing staff. Naturally, this meeting became a forum for the expression of condolences and not a review of the ethical issues in the case. However, because the nursing staff wanted guidance for similar situations in the future, one of the ethicists, with the assistance of two of the nurses involved, initiated a review by the IEC. The ethicist provided a summary of the conflicts:

> As I understood it, the patient [M] was near death. The physician had agreed with the family that the patient would be treated conservatively, that is, symptomatically—there would be no interventions like feeding tubes and that sort of thing—and that the patient would be kept "comfortable," which would include things like mouth care, turning, other nursing

care like that. The source of the problem seemed to be the family's insistence that the patient be given nothing by mouth even in the very final days and hours of [M's] dying. The concern—the family was informed by the physician that [M] had swallowing difficulties and [that there was a concern about aspiration]. The nurses' view, as I understood it, was that the mouth care that they would be providing would include things like ice chips, swabbing, sips of water, that sort of thing. [The nurses said] that [M] seemed to be pleading to have sips of water or drinks from the styrofoam cup, but that if there were family members present in the room, they insisted that nothing be given. [M] was in and out [of consciousness].

At one level, the nurses' ethical concerns were dismissed by distinguishing ethical issues from communication issues. This is a surprising distinction given the sensitivity to communication in two of the five "Terms of Reference" of the Rest Haven IEC: facilitating communication among staff, residents/patients, families, and the committee with respect to ethical issues, and maintaining communication between Rest Haven and the sisters' other facilities. But the reaction of one IEC member was typical: "I think that many on the committee were very upset that the issue even came to the committee. They were very upset that what to some was an ethical problem was, in fact, perceived by many to be just a difficult family problem—interpersonal conflicts between members of the family and different nursing staff—with no real ethical problem at the root of it. They just saw this as being an interpersonal communication problem."

The nurses' moral dilemma—do what they thought best for M given M's requests or abide by the wishes of M's family—was labeled a communication problem with no recognition that ethical controversies are deeply embedded in surrounding social processes, particularly those that involve communication. Here there was a clash between a family who did not want M to be given anything by mouth or tube and nurses who felt that M was sometimes conscious and pleading for water, a request that they had a moral obligation to fulfill. Whether the family and the nurses communicated their positions well or badly is a separate, but contextually connected, issue. The clash itself, though, was a weighty ethical dilemma worthy of the IEC's consideration. At the very least, it was an opportunity for the IEC to fulfill its educational mandate by recognizing the intimate relationship between ethics and communication and by promoting a deeper understanding of the most vexing ethical issue in long-term care—the withholding and withdrawal of nutrition and hydration. At most, it was an opportunity for everyone to reflect on the definitions of ethics and ethical principles they upheld and to expose and test those definitions in addressing this serious conflict.

At a deeper level, the dismissal of the nurses' dilemma can be traced to hierarchical and power relationships within the institution. The following quotations, the first from an administrator and the second from a physician, reveal that this case was not regarded as presenting ethical problems worthy of the IEC's review precisely because the dilemma was experienced by staff nurses:

> I think that, having been through the experience of having staff members [i.e., the nurses] bring a problem to the ethics committee, such access can be problematic because there's an assumption that every problem or dilemma is an ethical one, and I don't think that this serves well the people who are bringing the problem forward or the committee members themselves—to have to field those kinds of things. We have all kinds of other systems in place to make sure that problems on individual units can be dealt with. So I would be very reluctant to use the committee as a place to field dilemmas from specific groups of people.

> The nursing staff had difficulty accepting not feeding a patient. But they didn't [articulate that clearly]; and in fact, what happened there is that I heard comments about [the fact that] the patient was not on an NPO [i.e., nothing by mouth] order. I found this comment very comical, but they were very serious about it. They were dead serious that not having a physician ordering NPO meant that they had to feed the patient or, at least, offer food. The thing is that the family didn't want anything artificial. . . . NPO has a very medical meaning—it usually goes with specific medical or surgical interventions [but it wasn't relevant in this case]. I mean, it might be relevant from the nursing point of view—if there is an order, then they can be very clear on that—but what I don't accept is that having an NPO order on the chart would relieve the nurse of any moral questions. It might relieve the nurse of the legal responsibility, but not of the moral responsibility. . . . I personally was surprised [when the case went to the ethics committee] because from my point of view, it was such a clear-cut case. To me, the case did not present any ethical or moral problems. . . . I found that was a very interesting thing; the majority of the physicians who attended that meeting didn't have any problems with it; it was the nurses.

In this hierarchical rejection of the nurses' definition of the problem, the nurses' credibility was diminished by a phenomenon called "psychologizing"—the practice of dismissing people's behavior and views by interpreting them within a psychologistic framework (Anspach 1993:142–148). Through psychologizing, people "who disagree—rather than being seen as having their reasons, their values, and their life-plans—are seen as disturbed, subjects for psychological services" (Bosk 1998:112, n.5). In this Rest Haven situation, as so often happens when psychologizing occurs, the dismissal of the nurses' concerns was muted by apparent compliments. The following three reactions from IEC members illustrate this phenomenon, and the third goes beyond psychologizing to label the nurses' unit "dysfunctional":

> The nurses came to the committee and presented their case, which was highly emotional, of course, as well as concerned.

> It's a funny thing what happened there. I know those nurses. They're quite intelligent and collected people, and I wouldn't call them "emotional"; but they became very emotional during the meeting.

> About that particular case, I have sort of a bias about what goes on in that particular unit and when you listen to it, I was not alone in what I felt was happening. . . . It's characteristic of that particular unit. Not that they're not a good unit; they are; they're excellent people and devoted nurses. But someone on the committee said that it's obviously a dysfunctional unit. They were very protective of each other and the patient, but there was a real battle with families [i.e., historically]—maybe never as blatant as this one particular case. . . . Yet they're wonderful people; they're devoted nurses and they give good care; but they get themselves into these [presumably "dysfunctional"] situations, and they don't really bend in them.

But another IEC member insightfully recognizes what occurred:

> I think there's major problems because the structure of the organization—it's a systemic problem—it didn't disenfranchise—maybe that's too strong a word—somehow, the views of those nurses—somehow I felt they were marginalized in that whole enterprise. . . . Maybe they have a history of not working well with families—perhaps they do; but it seems to me that we all somehow discredit the perception of the bedside RNA [registered nursing assistant] as being unimportant. . . . They don't say that you have a legitimate point of view; they say, "You don't understand the problem." Well, people understand it only too well!! I see this in other feeding problems. . . . Why does the RNA believe that stopping feeding for a patient in a vegetative state is starving the patient to death when everybody else seems to be quite comfortable with discontinuing [the feeding]? . . . When there's real genuine ethical difference like that, [the nursing staff] have to be an integral part of the conversation about the question rather than saying to them paternalistically or patronizingly, "Well, you really don't understand what the problem is and if you did, there wouldn't be a problem." I'm sorry, but that's not very helpful!

The rejection of the nurses' views also featured stereotypical gender-specific notions that traditionally have degraded nurses, undermined their work, and made the development of higher education for nurses arduous. The nurses generally were not viewed as adult moral agents. In addition to being labeled "emotional," they were deprecated as "girls." The nurses were patronized also by comments that perpetuate the impression that women reside in the practical, not the intellectual, realm: "Let's face it, the majority of the nursing staff here have a—they are not very highly educated people. . . . They are very practical, very pragmatic. The majority of them are excellent people . . . but certainly not intellectuals."

Finally, there is a correspondence between the hierarchical division of labor within health care and hierarchically structured epistemologies or ways of knowing, and it seems to me that these parallel hierarchies also played a role in diminishing the nurses' dilemma. In the context of neonatal intensive care, Anspach (1993) found that physician-nurse disagreements about infants' prognoses could be attributed to a confrontation between three modes of knowing: the technological, the perceptual, and the interactive. Technological knowing relies on "hard" scientific evidence (e.g., as procured by diagnostic technology), which is more or less definitive in relation to the medical notions of "signs," "symptoms," and "disease." Perceptual knowing is based on data gathered by means such as palpation, percussion, and, most commonly, observation. Finally, interactive knowing arises out of social interaction, which includes both verbal and nonverbal communication. Anspach (1993) found that whereas all the occupational groups in the nurseries she studied engaged in the first two modes of knowing, a substantially larger number of nurses than physicians engaged in interactive knowing. Moreover, given the superior epistemological status ascribed to technological knowing, nurse-physician disagreements about prognosis were typically dominated by the physicians' technologically based assessments.

If we look again at the Rest Haven feeding case, physicians dismissed the nurses' concerns because in their view they were not ethical problems. This interpretation is understandable if we consider that on the level of technological and perceptual knowing, M was clearly incompetent and dying, "natural feeding" was virtually impossible, and the legitimate decisionmakers to whom the physicians were responsible, the family, had indicated that they did not want artificial feeding, the only remaining action that could have been ordered. Even an NPO order was out of the question because it had a specific technological and perceptual meaning, the requirements of which this patient did not meet (i.e., M was not a candidate for the medical or surgical interventions usually associated with an NPO order).

By contrast, that this situation created significant ethical problems for the nursing staff is understandable, too, because the information they obtained perceptually and interactively indicated that the patient was intermittently competent and able to express hunger in some way; that "natural feeding" was feasible to a limited degree and, at the very least, the desirability of such feeding could be assessed daily; and that, consequently, the family's decision and behavior created a conflict with the nurses' professional and moral obligations. The nurses had an obligation to care for M in accordance with their professional assessments and an obligation to uphold the facility's commitment to provide compassionate palliative care for dying patients. The nurses' collective sense of the importance of these obligations was clearly articulated by one of the nurses who cared for M:

> We were not uncomfortable feeding [M]. However, [a family member] had been feeding [M] one day and [M] choked [during this feeding]. This frightened [the family member who] didn't want to do it anymore. So a decision was made that [M] wouldn't be fed anymore. The staff were uncomfortable with that because they felt there were times when [M] could eat and also . . . on more than one occasion, [M] told the evening staff that [M] was hungry and they wanted to feed [M], but the family intervened. . . . It was very difficult because [M] was able to say that [M] wanted to eat. . . . However, [at the IEC meeting], the doctors said that [M] didn't really know what [M] was saying. . . . Our feeling was that there are probably cases where the patient should not be fed; but in this case, we felt that a daily assessment would have been better than making this decision which the family really didn't seem to understand because they really blocked anything being given by mouth. . . . There was a lot of assuming going on . . . that we were having trouble dealing with death and the way [M] died. . . . Let's face it, our patients do not get better and we've had to deal with a lot of death over the years. We know how to deal with that. . . . Maybe it wasn't clear to the family that when [a decision is made] not to feed a patient, that doesn't mean that we can't give [the patient] anything at all by mouth. . . . Maybe they should have been told that what we would do is assess [the situation] every day.

CONCLUSIONS

My data give credence to Storch and Griener's impression that IECs support existing institutional structures and power relationships. Although the terms of reference and access policy for Rest Haven's IEC created the potential to resolve ethical problems collegially at the local level, contextual factors seriously thwarted that potential. The IEC's status as a board committee resulted in a membership that was distanced from the bedside and that gave higher priority to risk management and public relations concerns than to the internal critique prompted by ethical reflection. Although confidentiality is essential for any IEC, preserving confidentiality complicated the Rest Haven IEC's attempts to receive input from front-line caregivers and to keep the facility informed about the overall ethics enterprise. The dichotomy between the IEC's theoretical/public and practical/private group identity was mirrored in the tension individual members personally experienced between their professional personae and their private vulnerability. As a result, ten years went by before a resident was allowed to become a member of the IEC.

Incompatible work schedules hampered access, particularly to the educational opportunities offered by the IEC. Most of all, access was impeded by the social processes and structures in which health care ethics is deeply embedded—notably, in this case, the gendered hierarchy of a hospital. Storch and Griener pondered why differences in ease of access occurred between physicians and nurses and "why the nurses might know so little about ethics committees." Inspired by and consistent with Anspach's analysis, my research also suggests that knowing about ethics and ethical knowing cannot be separated from the hierarchical, gendered processes through which all knowledge is created and organized in the clinical world.[4] These processes assign credibility to certain types of knowing (e.g., technological knowing) and render others (e.g., interactive knowing) less valuable. And as Anspach and others have documented, the less-valued types of knowing are attributed to the female gender. Ethics at Rest Haven was intimately bound up in these social processes.

With respect to the bigger question of whether IECs have fulfilled the expectations of the president's commission, I think the jury is still out. The experiences and hopes of the late 1970s and early 1980s inspired the commission's recommendations. Similar experiences and hopes prompted the creation of Rest Haven's IEC and ethics consultation service. Considering the medical paternalism that thrived previously, the commission's recommendations (especially those emphasizing diversity, contextual analysis, and community involvement) and the creation of Rest Haven's IEC are valiant changes. But whether these changes merely mask a more subtle, cautious paternalism, represent modest reform, or signify that systemic, consensual partnerships have displaced paternalism, is a question for this new millennium.

NOTES

Acknowledgments: I thank Renee Anspach, Michael Burgess, Barry Hoffmaster, and Barbara Koenig for their generous and helpful feedback as this chapter developed.

1. For empirical studies of IECs, see Avard, Griener, and Langstaff 1985; d'Oronzio, Dunn, and Gregory 1991; Flynn 1991; Hern 1990; Paré and Parizeau 1991; Scheirton 1992, 1993; Smith et al. 1992; Storch and Griener 1992; Storch et al. 1990; Wilson et al. 1993; Youngner et al. 1983, 1984. For empirical studies of ethics consultation, see Andereck 1992; Frader 1992; Griener and Storch 1994; Kelly et al. 1997; La Puma 1987; La Puma et al. 1988; Perkins and Saathoff 1988; Simpson 1992; Skeel and Self 1989.

2. For discussions of access problems, see Agich and Youngner 1991; Cohen and d'Oronzio 1989; Fost and Cranford 1985; Griener and Storch 1994; Handelsman 1995; Hoffman 1993; Mozdzierz, Reiquam, and Smith 1989; Nash, Leinbach, and Fought 1989.

3. "Rest Haven" is a pseudonym.

4. Although Chambliss (1996) does not deal directly with gendered epistemologies and their implications in nursing, he does provide valuable insights into the connection between nurses' work and femininity as structured in the clinic and beyond, for example, "The structure of the work reinforces and supports the going conceptions of femininity in the larger society, and this is not lost on people choosing (or not) a career in nursing" (1996:84).

REFERENCES

Agich, George J., and Stuart J. Youngner. 1991. For Experts Only? Access to Hospital Ethics Committees. *Hastings Center Report* 21(5):17–25.

Allatt, Peter, and Meg Sheehan. 1992. Ethics Committees: Promoting Effectiveness—Preventing Dysfunction. *Canadian Health Care Management* April:ET 5.1–5.9.

Andereck, William S. 1992. Development of a Hospital Ethics Committee: Lessons from Five Years of Case Consultations. *Cambridge Quarterly of Healthcare Ethics* 1:41–50.

Anspach, Renee R. 1993. *Deciding Who Lives: Fateful Choices in the Intensive-Care Nursery*. Berkeley: University of California Press.

Avard, D., G. Griener, and J. Langstaff. 1985. Hospital Ethics Committees: Survey Reveals Characteristics. *Dimensions of Health Service* 62(2):24–26.

Bosk, Charles L., and Joel Frader. 1998. Institutional Ethics Committees: Sociological Oxymoron, Empirical Black Box. In *Bioethics and Society: Constructing the Ethical Enterprise*, eds. Raymond DeVries and Janardan Subedi, 94–116. Upper Saddle River, NJ: Prentice Hall.

Chambliss, Daniel F. 1996. *Beyond Caring: Hospitals, Nurses, and the Social Organization of Ethics*. Chicago: University of Chicago Press.

Cohen, C. J., and J. C. d'Oronzio. 1989. The Question of Access. *HEC Forum* 1:89–103.

d'Oronzio, J. C., D. Dunn, and J. J. Gregory. 1991. A Survey of New Jersey Hospital Ethics Committees. *HEC Forum* 3:255–268.

Flynn, P. A. 1991. *Moral Ordering and the Social Construction of Bioethics*. Ph.D. Thesis, University of California, San Francisco.

Fost, Norman, and R. E. Cranford. 1985. Hospital Ethics Committees: Administrative Aspects. *Journal of the American Medical Association* 253:2687–2697.

Frader, Joel E. 1992. Political and Interpersonal Aspects of Ethics Consultation. *Theoretical Medicine* 13:31- 44.

Griener, Glenn G., and J. L. Storch. 1994. The Educational Needs of Ethics Committees. *Cambridge Quarterly of Healthcare Ethics* 3:467–477.

Handelsman, M. M. 1995. Canaries in the Mine Shaft: Frustrations and Benefits of Community Members on Ethics Committees. *HEC Forum* 7:278–283.

Hern, H. Gene. 1990. Ethics and Human Values Committee Survey: A Study of Physician Attitudes and Perceptions of a Hospital Ethics Committee. *HEC Forum* 2:105–125.

Hoffman, D. E. 1993. Evaluating Ethics Committees: A View from the Outside. *Milbank Quarterly* 71:677- 701.

Holland, Joe, and Peter Henriot. 1989. *Social Analysis: Linking Faith and Justice*. Washington, DC: The Center of Concern.

Kelly, Susan E., Patricia A. Marshall, Lee M. Sanders, Thomas A. Raffin, and Barbara A. Koenig. 1997. Understanding the Practice of Ethics Consultation: Results of an Ethnographic Multi-Site Study. *Journal of Clinical Ethics* 8: 136–149.

La Puma, John. 1987 Consultations in Clinical Ethics—Issues and Questions in 27 Cases. *Western Journal of Medicine* 146:633–637.

La Puma, John, Carol B. Stocking, Marc D. Silverstein, Andrea DiMartini, and Mark Siegler. 1988. An Ethics Consultation Service in a Teaching Hospital: Utilization and Evaluation. *Journal of the American Medical Association* 260: 808–811.

Mozdzierz, G. J., C. W. Reiquam, and L. C. Smith. 1989. Shaping Access to Hospital Ethics Committees: Some Critical Issues. *HEC Forum* 1:31–39.

Mount, Eric. 1990. *Professional Ethics in Context: Institutions, Images and Empathy*. Louisville, KY: Westminster/John Knox.

Nash, R. B., M. L. Leinbach, and R. J. Fought. 1989. The Hospital Ethics Committee: Who Knows It Exists and How to Access It? *HEC Forum* 1:9–30.

Paré, S., and M.-H. Parizeau. 1991. Hospital Ethics Committees in Quebec: An Overview. *HEC Forum* 3:339–346.

Perkins, Henry S., and Bunnie S. Saathoff. 1988. Impact of Medical Ethics Consultations on Physicians: An Exploratory Study. *American Journal of Medicine* 85:761–765.

President's Commission for the Study of Ethical Problems in Medicine and Biomedical and Behavioral Research. 1983. *Deciding to Forego Life-Sustaining Treatment.* Washington, DC: U.S. Government Printing Office.

Scheirton, Linda S. 1992. Determinants of Hospital Ethics Committee Success. *HEC Forum* 4:342–359.

———. 1993. Measuring Hospital Ethics Committee Success. *Cambridge Quarterly of Healthcare Ethics* 2:495–504.

Simpson, Kenneth H. 1992. The Development of a Clinical Ethics Consultation Service in a Community Hospital. *Journal of Clinical Ethics* 3:124–130.

Skeel, Joy D., and Donnie J. Self. 1989. An Analysis of Ethics Consultation in the Clinical Setting. *Theoretical Medicine* 10:289–299.

Smith, Martin, Janet Day, Robert Collins, and Gerald Erenberg. 1992. A Survey on Awareness and Effectiveness of Bioethics Resources. *HEC Forum* 4:1 87–197.

Storch, Janet L., and Glenn G. Griener. 1992. Ethics Committees in Canadian Hospitals: Report of the 1990 Pilot Study. *Healthcare Management FORUM* 5(1):19–26.

Storch, Janet L., Glenn G. Griener, Deborah A. Marshall, and Beverly A. Olineck. 1990. Ethics Committees in Canadian Hospitals: Report of the 1989 Survey. *Healthcare Management FORUM* 3(4):3–8.

Wilson, Robin Fretwell, Martha Neff-Smith, Donald Phillips, and John C. Fletcher. 1993. HECs: Are They Evaluating Their Performance? *HEC Forum* 5:1–34.

Youngner, Stuart J., Claudia Coulton, Barbara W. Juknialis, and David L. Jackson. 1984. Patients' Attitudes toward Hospital Ethics Committees. *Law, Medicine & Health Care* 12:21–25.

Youngner, Stuart J., David L. Jackson, Claudia Coulton, Barbara W. Juknialis, and Era M. Smith. 1983. A National Survey of Hospital Ethics Committees. *Critical Care Medicine* 11:902–905.

CHARLES L. BOSK

9   Irony, Ethnography, and Informed Consent

MUCH OF this volume is an argument for and demonstration of two interrelated propositions: Bioethical analysis can be made sharper if more attention is paid to the context of medical decision making, and ethnography is the ideal method for accomplishing this. Intellectual completeness and honesty—not to mention the self-reflexive dimension of ethnographic work itself—require that attention to the ethnography of medical ethics be matched by a reciprocal analysis of the ethics of ethnography.

That is the task of this chapter. In it, I first discuss some of the standard ethical dilemmas fieldworkers recognize as inherent in ethnographic methods. Here, I argue that the commonly rehearsed ethical dilemmas of fieldwork screen our attention from some more fundamental problems of fieldwork, especially when that work is among highly literate subjects within one's own culture. Then, using my own fieldwork among surgeons, genetic counselors, and workers in a pediatric intensive care unit as an example, I discuss these primary, and perhaps irresolvable, ethical problems of ethnography.

Such an analysis is necessary for two major reasons. First, it will avoid the inevitable disappointment that occurs when an idea is pushed beyond its serviceable boundaries. Ethnography—and other forms of social science research—have a place in bioethics. They are useful in providing answers to some sorts of questions and concerns but not to others. It is important to be clear about these limits. Ethnographers need to take care not to promise, and bioethicists not to expect, too much from a labor-intensive mode of inquiry that is highly dependent on the individual researcher's subjectivity, sensitivity, and interpersonal skills; that is useful for describing social process in very specific circumstances but not for generalizing across settings; and that has no way to describe values and beliefs other than as reflections of socially structured interests with no independent ontological status of their own.

Next, traditionally ethnographies have been done by ethnographers who occupy specific niches in social science departments, have received training in concrete intellectual traditions, and have very definite value commitments regarding the purposes of their work. Bioethicists occupy different occupational roles, receive a different training, and possess, as a rule, different value commitments. How well these two distinct sets of roles, training, and value commitments harmonize is an open question. I argue below that excellence in one domain—ethnography—may make excellence in the other—bioethics—difficult, if not impossible. At the very least, the doctrine of "fully informed voluntary consent" requires that bioethicists be aware of the risks and benefits of embracing ethnographic research, in particular, and social science methods, more generally.

Throughout this discussion, I point out some pragmatic difficulties in either creating or using ethnographic accounts as part of the academic literature of bioethics or the public discourse of the ethical dilemmas of medicine. For the purposes of furthering a discussion of *ethics*, ethnography, despite its superficial allure, is not ideal. The description is just too detailed; and if it is not, then the ethnography is inadequate, an unreliable basis on which to found an argument. The goal of ethnographic analysis is not to clarify on which values action should be bottomed. Rather, the goal is to show how flexible values are, how the same values are used to justify a wide range of seemingly incompatible behaviors. But there are other reasons for ethicists to be wary of ethnography. A close look at the methods used to generate ethnographic data and to produce ethnographic accounts raises questions that suggest that these research tools have insuperable ethical problems in terms of informed consent and the preservation of confidentiality and anonymity. These necessary moral failings are built into the structure of ethnographic research. This fact might give the ethicist pause before using the insights generated by such suspect behaviors. That these problems are largely unacknowledged becomes clear when we review the traditional approach ethnographers take to the ethical problems that they recognize as part of their research methods.

EVERYDAY ETHICS OF ETHNOGRAPHY

For its first sociological practitioners, primary observation of social life was not problematic either methodologically or ethically. In the sustained body of urban studies produced during the 1920s and 1930s, the sociologists of the Chicago School studied the city as "a mosaic of social life" (Park and Burgess [1922] 1967). A key advocate of this approach, Robert Park, a former reporter, emphasized in his programmatic writing the connection between the physical and moral space of the city. The early monographs that the Chicago School produced all tended to be structured along very similar lines—a "natural" area of the city is identified; the demographic, geographic, and economic features of this unique "ecological" niche are specified through summary statistics; and, then, on the basis of observation and in situ interviewing, the "moral order" of the "natural" area is described. None of the authors of these studies raise any questions about the observational data. Valid data required only an observer with a notebook.

Questions about ethnographic methods begin within sociology, like so much else, with the publication of the second edition of William Foote Whyte's *Street Corner Society* (1955). Whyte reports that when *Street Corner Society* first appeared in 1943, its commercial success was underwhelming. Brisk sales came only with the revised, expanded second edition, which includes a methodological appendix that explains how the research was done. There are a number of reasons why the second edition was so much more commercially successful than the first. In part, the new appendix makes for a more artful presentation and for a more "real" account. But demographic and cultural considerations played a role as well. When college enrollments began expanding, there was a need within sociology for an accessible text to engage students. Also, in the war years the concerns of *Street Corner Society*—the assimilation and resistance of the sons of Italian American immigrants to mainstream American society—must have seemed far away. Oddly, the passage of time allowed for the subject matter to become more timely. Finally, Whyte's themes resonated with many of the ongoing themes of the civil rights movement and permitted their discussion absent race, which, undoubtedly, must have made the discourse more comfortable for a while at least.

Since Whyte, such appendices are a standard part of ethnographic writing—so much so that Van Maanen (1988) in his survey of ethnographic writing identifies them as a distinct subgenre that he labeled "confessionals." Although Van Maanen's label has a trivializing connotation—think ethnographers on Oprah or Sally Jesse Raphael—it is also surprisingly apt.

There is a sense in which one thing that all ethnographers do in appendices is ask their colleagues' forgiveness for various sins against method idealized. In Whyte's first-ever example of what was later to become so stylized, he described what over time became the commonly rehearsed issues of participant observation with their standard solutions. The most important of these are as follows: the difficulties of gaining entry to a setting, of winning the trust of one's subjects, of balancing obligations to competing groups within the neighborhood, of verifying one's own insights about what is going on, and of leaving the setting.

From Whyte's appendix, we learn of his settling into Cornerville; of his meeting "Doc"; of his continual struggles to fit into the alien neighborhood of Cornerville; and of his initial indifference, then his excitement, and finally his horror at voting numerous times in a local election. This last revelation is a touchstone for confessional ethnographic writing. Whyte reports being troubled by this ethical lapse only when threatened with public exposure and disgrace. However much Whyte strains to sound concerned by his ethical lapse, his account conveys nothing so much as his excitement at being accepted and trusted enough to engage in this conventional political petty larceny.

Although there are a number of things worth noting about this report of the fieldworker's dilemma, one thing that is not is its resolution: to follow local customs, to go native. In fact, examples of instances in which the researcher behaved in ways that violated his or her everyday norms are easy to multiply. It is hard to imagine how it could be otherwise. After all, sociologists report being drawn to settings "where the action is," and the scene of ethically problematic activities is just one such setting (Goffman 1961). This is as true of the street corner and its petty crimes as it is of the intensive care unit with its ineluctable treatment dilemmas. One could hardly study such issues if one responded moralistically—to learn about fences requires knowledge of stolen goods (Klockars 1974), to study youth gangs involves observing street violence (Sanchez-Jankowski 1991), to observe how welfare recipients get by on limited incomes means keeping an open mind about what officials label welfare fraud (Edin and Lein 1997), to study decision making in intensive care demands suspending judgments about how such judgments ought to be made (Anspach 1993; Zussman 1992), and to catalogue medical error from the physician's point of view asks that other points of view be submerged (Bosk 1979).

In fact, when ethnographers evaluate their behavior in the field, they rarely use an ethical yardstick. Instead, they use a pragmatic one. The question is not whether the act in question violated everyday norms. Rather, the question posed is, Did the questionable behavior contribute to doing the study? With this kind of moral accounting, most actions, however far beyond the pale they are, are justified easily. But there is something self-serving in this. Ethnography is not a carefully controlled clinical experiment; the fieldworker never knows for sure what the consequences of acting alternatively would have been, never knows if the boundaries could have been drawn differently. This mode of moral accounting does, however, draw attention to a central facet of being in the field: The pressure to fit in, go along, suspend disbelief, and discount one's own moral autonomy in the name of research is enormous and, perhaps sadly, irresistible.

Nowhere in the writing about doing the research is the pragmatic stance of the fieldworker and its distance from a moral one so clearly marked as in discussions about gaining entry. In appendical musings, ethnographers recount their worries about fashioning plausible cover stories to explain their interest and presence in a field setting. A good cover story provides an easily understood rationale, but is not so overly detailed that it distorts later responses, creating dreaded "observer" effects. Many discussions of telling cover stories have a "comical aspect" (for a good example, see Bluebond-Langer 1978). In the typical account, the fieldworker reports great apprehension, a carefully prepared speech clumsily delivered, and, finally, the irrelevance of both the worry and the story itself. In the end, entry and trust are negotiated and renegotiated over time. What matters is not what is said once and formally, but what is done repeatedly and spontaneously.

Drawing on my own experience, I would place very bold quotation marks around the word "spontaneously." When I am in the field, very little ever feels spontaneous to me. Rather, I am constantly calculating and weighing responses in terms of the kind of data they are likely to yield in both the long and short run. To be sure, this is an instantaneous calculation in which I am most probably frequently wrong. Nonetheless, my responses are based on this; they are calculations, not spontaneous expressions of my most authentic, innermost self. The very fact that this is so causes me to wonder if ethnographers' understanding of observer effects is not as self-serving as their rationales for norm violations. Ethnographers acknowledge that observer effects rarely can be gauged directly from first-hand observations. Ethnographers cannot make observations of how group members behave when the ethnographer is absent. Then, ethnographers argue that in the face of natural role demands and situational exigencies, observer effects disappear over time, are minimal, or both. This is an argument that has considerable appeal, allowing, as it does, ethnographers to discount any impact they might have had on that which they describe.

This is an argument in which I once fervently believed—but lately, like some turn-of-the-century cleric exposed to Ingersoll, I have come to have my doubts. As I look over what I have observed, thought I understood, and interpreted authoritatively, I wonder how much was staged for my benefit. I have been blessed and cursed with "theatrical" natives with more than enough savvy to figure out my interests. Those disciplinings that modeled the surgical conscience (Bosk 1979), and those tortured, quasi-religious meditations on the ethics of genetics and its applications (Bosk 1992)—how genuine were they really? Might they have not taken place if I had been absent and subjects felt no obligation to show just how seriously they took those obligations in which I was most interested? I did not much entertain these doubts at the time of the fieldwork. The data were often too good to question in this way. But now I wonder if I need to reconsider how an attentive audience of one with a tape recorder or stenographer's notebook, taking down every word, might cause a self-conscious subject to play his or her social role "over the top." Because such role performances make the task of the ethnographer so much easier, ethnographers have little incentive for asking these questions in this way. In fact, incentives run the other way, leading researchers to dismiss the possibility of such observer effects. But if I am able to sustain my role performance for the duration of the fieldwork, why is the same not true of those who are observed?

Questions of observer effect aside, it is worth returning to "cover stories" and paying attention to what they do not discuss and what ethnographers avoid discussing up-front. First, for methodological reasons, ethnographers obscure or keep vague their research questions. Next, ethnographers do not discuss what the experience of being observed might be like for subjects. Subjects who are curious or apprehensive about the impact of observation routinely are assured that impacts are benign, that the researcher is just one more "hale fellow well met," who would never, ever, interfere with the ongoing group process. Researchers assume that subjects who wish to avoid observation will find ways to do so. We certainly feel little obligation to spell out a subject's right not to participate. We routinely promise confidentiality and anonymity, but we do not discuss how this promise is easy to make but difficult to fulfill.

I do not mean to imply that ethnographers do not take moral obligations seriously. The literature provides a fairly standardized corpus of ethical questions, spectacular examples of questionable behavior in the past, and a lively debate about our professional responsibilities. For example, to preserve confidentiality, ethnographers have accepted incarceration. This certainly is evidence of serious moral commitment. By the same token, to gather data otherwise unobtainable, ethnographers have conducted covert observations and then worried in their texts about the appropriateness of doing so. Ethnographers have endangered themselves for their subjects; and they have, unwittingly, endangered their subjects in their publications. None of these are topics that a researcher worried about access and entry would choose to mention to a potential but reluctant research subject. All of this suggests nothing less than that the world is a morally complex place. This is not news. What I wish to point out here is something else: Our sociological imagination has been dulled by repeatedly grinding it against the same issues. Fieldwork is more morally complex than the constant rehearsal of the same issues suggests. In general, our discussions of rapport, of confidentiality, of the codes of conduct for researchers evade rather than confront the moral complexities of fieldwork. It is this subject to which I now turn.

ETHNOGRAPHY AS A MORALLY PROBLEMATIC ACTIVITY

As a human activity, fieldwork is most peculiar because it contravenes so many of the ordinary rules of everyday social life. It is not just that researchers who do fieldwork watch social life as it unfolds and then report on it, in the process airing much of a group's dirty linen (although we ethnographers do that for certain); it is not just that ethnographers take a group's most cherished notions of itself and show how these are self-serving (although we do that for certain as well); rather, it is how ethnographers do these things that makes fieldwork sometimes feel like such a morally dubious human activity. The key word here is human. Fieldwork is, whatever its difficulties, often redeemed by the fact that it is a human activity. It involves living with and coming to know a group of "strangers." Other research methods are not quite so humanly involving. Of field methods, I feel as others may feel about democracy—it is a terrible method; it is just better (for the kinds of questions that intrigue me) than all the alternatives. This, more than anything else, allows me to engage in the multiple morally dubious behaviors described below.

First, ethnographers trade quite freely on an almost universal misunderstanding between our research subjects and ourselves. For most subjects, the opportunity to be studied is flattering: It feeds or confirms a sense of specialness; it is a vehicle for being lifted out of the ordinary and everyday; and it is even seen by some as a backdoor to an obscure, academic immortality. Because our subjects are flattered by our attention, we are allowed to obtain data that it is not necessarily in our subjects' best interest to reveal. Few of us have ever reported that we inform our subjects of this fact. Rather, because it so often serves our purposes so well, we encourage any misperceptions that yield rich data.

Exactly what makes data rich, what allows data to sustain a "thick description" (Geertz 1973), is hard to specify absent a concrete situation. However, a rule of thumb is easy to provide: Rich data subvert official definitions, generally accepted public understandings, and conventional wisdom. Such data tell us what public records and official statistics conceal. Such data are best gathered backstage, behind the yellow tape and the sign limiting access to authorized personnel. Above all, rich data are data that allow the observer the opportunity to interpret social life ironically.

In so doing, we ethnographers betray our subjects twice: first, when we manipulate our relationship with subjects to generate data and then again when we retire to our desks to transform experience to text. This second betrayal is the one my subjects have felt the most keenly. It is the one about which they have complained. Whether it causes them to reevaluate the quasi-friendship we had during the time I was conducting the fieldwork, I do not know (and, in truth, would probably prefer not to know). Both surgeons and genetic counselors felt misrepresented by my attempts to provide what I—but not they—considered an objective description of their occupational world. This sense of betrayal did not center on the accuracy of my description. Both surgeons and genetic counselors agreed that things had happened as I had described them.

Their sense of betrayal centered on the contexts within which I placed the description of incidents rather than the incidental description itself.

After reviewing my manuscript for *Forgive and Remember* (1979), the chair of surgery objected to my framing my discussion of mistakes in a sociological rhetoric borrowed from the vocabulary of deviance and social control. He felt, and he let me know that a number of other attendings who had also read the manuscript also felt, that this language was entirely inappropriate: Surgery was too noble a profession for this treatment. He suggested that he, and those other nonspecified colleagues who shared his concern and with whom he had discussed the problem, would prefer a discussion in terms of suboptimal performance rather than mistakes. He and his colleagues felt that all this talk of deviance obscured the background of excellence against which the incidents I described so accurately—and here there was a mixture of flattery and amazement in his tone—came to be thought of as mistakes. I told him that I appreciated his and his colleagues' concerns, that I was grateful for the places in the text where they corrected technical details and misspellings to rescue me from embarrassment, that I was happy to remove an offending phrase here or a too revealing detail there, but that was all. The sociological interpretation was my business, not his. It was the domain where I was the expert. It was his and his colleagues' life but my interpretation. He was not happy. We were both surprised by my assertion of authorial privilege, given the differences in age and rank between us. But, somewhat grudgingly, he yielded—it was my interpretation, after all; and there was still some question in both our minds as to whether it would ever see the light of day.

The same issue of interpretive license arose after my informants read a prepublication version of *All God's Mistakes* (1992). I remember dropping the text off at the office of the genetic counselor who in the text is known as Bill Smith. He received the text with what seemed to be genuine joy—a huge grin followed by a warm hug—at my having completed a much-delayed project. As I waited, Bill, with a new assistant whom I had just met, began to leaf through the text, starting with the table of contents. Joy quickly turned to a mixture of horror, fear, and disapproval. "'A Mop-Up Service, Janitors, Shock Absorbers.' . . . Oh no . . . Bosk, you can't say this," said Bill. The assistant responded, "But why not, you say it every day." Bill told her, "That's different. I say it to you, to the walls of my office, to the conference room. It's one thing for

you all to know what I think. It's another to put it out there for everyone to see. How will I work with these people?"

I thought at the time that Bill Smith's reaction encapsulated all that
had made him such an interesting subject: an over-the-top, on-his-
sleeve, quickly verbalized emotional reaction to an unexpected situation. Such responses were as transient as they were entertaining. I
expected Bill to adjust. I was wrong. Late that afternoon when I
returned to my office there was a call from the hospital attorney of
Nightingale Children's Hospital. She informed me that Bill Smith was
very upset and had called her to discuss the possibility of blocking publication. I asked, "On what grounds?" She said that Smith and the others in the work group felt that their identities were not blinded
sufficiently. As a result, they felt that the work "held them up to public
ridicule and irreparably harmed their professional reputations." In
addition, the lawyer stated, all of my subjects claimed to be unaware
that I was doing the research for the purpose of writing a book. Or, alternatively, they claimed (and at this point in the conversation, I was having some difficulty sorting out exactly what was being said, and even
with very precise notes am having some difficulty reconstructing it
now) that they thought I was studying patients and not the professional
staff. Therefore, I had gained these data without their fully informed
consent. Finally, they claimed to be worried about patient confidentiality, and, because I had not received formal consent to either observe ses-
sions or interview patients, I could not publish the data.

My first response was pugnacious. I suggested to the attorney that if
my subjects wanted to turn an obscure academic treatise into a First
Amendment issue, that was fine with me—I could hardly hope to get so
much free publicity any other way. The lawyer attempted to soothe me.
She told me that that was just the sort of thing she wanted to avoid, that
these physicians had thought of me as their friend and now they felt
betrayed (a feeling with which she agreed, given her quick skim of the
manuscript), and that she was offering her services to broker an amica-
ble settlement. She asked if I could let her know when I would be available over the next few days for a meeting.

After a few phone calls back and forth, we agreed that I was to meet
with my former friends and research subjects who were now my current adversaries the next morning. I spent a troubled night. Because the
research proposal from which the manuscript grew had been submitted

originally as part of a National Institutes of Health "Center" grant, the claim that my subject/informants had not known that they were the object of my attention was clearly not correct. My institution's institutional review board had approved the actual study; I had a drawerful of consent forms. I felt that all of my former friends' complaints were baseless. Yet, I also understood that the literal truth was not the most critical issue here. The more I thought about it—and try as I might I could not think of anything else—the more anxious I was, even though I knew bruised feelings were a "natural" part of good fieldwork. I had been taught that, in making the latent manifest, the fieldworker made his or her subjects uncomfortable. And I was also taught that this discomfort, which was likened to resistance in psychoanalytic theory, indicated that the ethnographic interpretation had some substance: An account that did not make subjects squirm was suspect, because it showed that the researcher had not penetrated deeply enough into the social world being described. What I had been taught, I was now teaching to my graduate students. Cognitively, I knew what they meant. I even understood that such beliefs served to protect fieldworkers emotionally by providing a rationale for understanding and then dismissing subjects' negative reactions to our work. However, I had never been brought face-to-face with the consequences of this belief system. It was an educational experience I would have preferred to avoid.

But that was not an option. So, there I was that next morning, sitting across from folks whose social world I long ago shared but who were now strangers—very angry strangers. And really there was more to it than that. As I discussed in *All God's Mistakes* (1992), I was invited by the genetic counselors to study them and their social world. They wanted help as they entered socially uncharted waters. They asked for help and what they felt they got instead was public humiliation. I had always been aware of this as a possible outcome. My fears about this, in fact, slowed the writing of this volume. It was a task I avoided for many years until all the junior colleagues involved in the fieldwork had either been promoted or not. Although I always realized that one consequence of the writing would be to confront some very hurt colleagues, I always assumed that such confrontations would be unplanned, would take place on social occasions, and would be contained by those occasions.

I never expected to confront colleagues in a meeting called specifically so that they could tell me exactly how badly I had wronged them.

On the advice of a friend and colleague at the University of Pennsylvania Law School, I brought along two observers. Because there were going to be three of my former colleagues present, my friend thought I ought to have an equal number of allies in the room. This way if there were a dispute later about what we agreed to, it would not simply be a matter of my word against theirs. My observers played no role in the subsequent negotiations, although they did provide comfort and support. Their presence was objected to by my former colleagues, but, at my insistence, they remained.

The meeting began with Bill Smith saying that he wished to read a statement. He needed to read the statement, he said, because he was worried that if he just spoke, he would not be able to control himself. He was so mad at me that he had not really thought he would be able to be in the same room with me—a written statement, he said, would let him say what he wanted to say the way he wanted to say it. Bill began to read in a quavering voice—it was clear that he was close to tears—and he was able to get through half his statement before he threw it on the table, turned to one of his colleagues and said simply, "finish," and left the room sobbing.

The statement, as I recall it, was a model of simple eloquence. Bill asserted that he had not slept since reading the manuscript, that he had always been proud of his work, that my work destroyed everything that he had accomplished, that I had in essence done nothing less than erase twenty years of professional achievements, that all of this was harder for him to take because he had always considered me a friend and because he was going through a difficult time in his life, and that if I had even a shard of decency left, I would not publish this book. He was begging me as one human being to another not to publish this book. The colleague who was reading Bill's words looked up after this closing request and said with simple understatement, "I guess you can tell that Bill is pretty upset. We're all a little put out. But the rest of us will get over it. But you have a problem with Bill."

I said that I could see that. I also said that they all should realize that not publishing was not an option. I went on to point out that no one had yet claimed that the book had any misrepresentation of what I had observed. The colleague assured me that what was disturbing, in part, was the accuracy of the description coupled with interpretations with which they did not agree. I said that I was willing to work with them so that the final version of the book made them all less identifiable. However,

I would not negotiate without Bill in the room. The colleague promised me that Bill would be present. (This was promised with an aside, "You remember how emotional Bill can be. We'll make sure he is here.")

A few more meetings and we reached an accord. It was a simple thing: A pseudonym here and there was changed to confuse gender and ethnicity. Some of the identifying details of Nightingale Hospital were misstated. (The hospital attorney asked me to change the bed number. It mattered little to her if I inflated or deflated the figure—either would do, as long as it was inaccurate.) I was asked to change a few rare diseases so patient confidentiality would not be compromised. The genetic counselors were helpful in identifying other rare disorders with the same risk of recurrence, mode of inheritance, and likelihood of prenatal diagnosis. We haggled a bit over some interpretive terms such as "mop-up service." But my line in the sand held firm: If the details were wrong, I would change them; if the details threatened to breach confidentiality and anonymity, I would blur them; if any extraneous remark, an aside in the flow of interaction, was likely to raise hackles unnecessarily, I would remove it; but the interpretation was, rightly or wrongly, for better or worse, mine.

Not surprisingly, this is the stance that has a great deal of legitimacy in an institution such as the modern tertiary care hospital, where professional turf and authority routinely are challenged and defended. That it is built out of a largely illusory distinction, that it is not so easy to disentangle facts from interpretive frameworks, that the authorial privilege, which I claimed rested on an expertise that is easily questioned—none of these issues were raised. Nor was a more troubling issue raised—that the sense of betrayal of the genetic counselors of Nightingale Children's Hospital, similar to that of the surgeons of Pacific Hospital before them, rested on a quite firm basis in reality. I had in some larger sense operated without informed consent. I had violated confidentiality and anonymity. Beyond that, these breaches were both inescapable and reasonably foreseeable. In fact, I believe it is impossible to do hospital-based ethnography without both violating informed consent and without breaking promises made to subjects about confidentiality and anonymity.

There is a trivial sense in which ethnographers cannot help but operate without informed consent. As strangers come and go in the environment, we cannot break up the flow of interaction to tell each newcomer that they have just entered a "research zone," that their words are likely to be recorded, and that their actions may be described and interpreted in a text at a later date. An overly scrupulous approach to informed consent would create disruptions of social life, would be intrusive, would heighten self-consciousness of actors to a high degree, and would be so socially bizarre that it would make fieldwork impossible to complete. But I think that this is something everyone recognizes and that no one expects every person who enters the field to be informed that they have just become an extra in someone else's social drama. However, there is a deeper level at which we breach the spirit of informed consent. We mislead subjects about our intentions and keep them in the dark about reasonable and easily recognized risks, even when our subjects understand (and misunderstand) our role—when they tell us, "I see, you're Malinowski and we are the Trobrianders," or when they inform us of their willingness to be subjects: "Oh yes, how we manage uncertainty, how we handle mistakes, how we define professional service, how we cope with pressure and stress—those are interesting questions. Of course, you can observe." We describe our intent, but we omit a detail. We disclose but only incompletely.

What we leave out is more important than what we choose to reveal. Of all that goes unsaid, the most important element is the hardest to explain, yet at the same time, it is fundamental for understanding the feelings of betrayal that subjects and informants so routinely experience. Subjects, being human, are flattered by our attention. Subjects, especially physicians in bureaucratic organizations, often feel beleaguered by demands from both patients and hospital administration. A common complaint is that dedicated service is unappreciated. A common sentiment is that if only the nature of the pressures on harried doctors were really understood, if only the complexities of the work were truly known, and if only the self-sacrifice were more visible, then physicians would receive more of the public esteem that many in the occupation feel they deserve but currently are denied. It is these negative sentiments and their potential correction—this sense of being chronically misunderstood—that fieldworkers tap into when they seek access to medical settings. Into this situation the ethnographer walks and tells his or her subjects, who feel so misunderstood, what they most want to hear. What the fieldworker promises to describe and explain—the subjects' world from the subject's point of view—is the story most subjects want desperately to have told. Physicians who know the social science literature, and they are not so numerous as one might hope, know that their wishes here may outrun reality. They may intuit that being understood is more than they can hope for, but a number of powerful forces countervail: The support for inquiry in academic medical centers and the lack of alternatives for having their stories told are two of the most important.

There would be nothing wrong with this if all or most of what we were interested in was the "world from the actors' point of view." But that is not the case, regardless of our disclaimers to the contrary. All good fieldwork must describe the "world from the actor's point of view," must record accurately what Geertz (1973) calls "the said" of social life, but this is the starting point—a necessary but not a sufficient element in producing adequate ethnography. Ethnographers do not inform subjects that the world from their point of view is the starting point for our interpretive activities. It is through these interpretations that subjects feel the sense of betrayal at ethnographic portraits of their social world. And this is not surprising because what is most unsettling to subjects about ethnographic interpretations is built into the way social scientists are socialized to think about the world.

The most characteristic ways a social scientist learns to think are organized to disabuse any group of its own notions of its "specialness." Social science is a generalizing activity. One implication of this is that when group members claim special qualities, sensitivities, skills, or privileges, ethnographers dutifully record these sentiments. We take the sacred beliefs of a group about itself seriously but not literally; and social scientists do more. We point out how such sentiments are shared by other groups and are manipulated by those groups for their own advantage; we show how altruistic beliefs cloak self-interest. In short, what we do is take a group's sense of its specialness and inspect it; and while inspecting it, we show how ordinary, commonplace, and self-serving it really is. Few groups are grateful for this.

What in all of this violates the spirit of informed consent? At the simplest level, I suppose it is no more complicated than this. Experienced ethnographers know that nothing is so prized in the social science literature as the counterintuitive finding, that no voice is so cultivated as the ironic, and that no spirit characterizes work so much as a debunking one. Yet we certainly do not warn our subjects of this. One might say that this is trivial—there is risk in all of this, but the harm is negligible. I am not so sure. I lost my certitude in the harmlessness of my methods and of my ways of describing them to my subjects on the morning Bill Smith tossed his written statement on the table and fled the room crying.

One might argue that, even if the risks of irony were explained, subjects would not be able to understand them; they would consent anyway and still feel betrayed in the end. After all, we social scientists expect to see the world from the subject's point of view, but we have the benefit of extensive professional training. How can we expect our subjects to intuit our objectives, to see the world clearly from our point of view? These are not arguments that are given much credence when physicians use them as an excuse for failing to provide patients the data necessary for informed consent. They possess no more credence when given by social scientists as a justification for less than full disclosure. The simple fact is that we do not try to explain this aspect of our work to our subjects, and we feel no obligation to try for this level of consent. The simplest explanation is that such disclosure is difficult; it does indeed impede our ability to gather our data and do our work. If this is the case, then these difficulties need to be confronted. Pretending that they do not exist is not an adequate response for the social scientist or any other researcher.

But there is another reason we do not feel duty-bound to disclose to subjects that ultimately they will feel betrayed by our ethnographic reports. The act of betrayal occurs after we have left the field. It occurs when we are no longer engaged with our subjects and when we no longer need their cooperation. Moreover, few of us are ever confronted by the egos our work bruises, the souls it lacerates, or the communal relationships it roils. This aspect of our work is not something we see, something we have to live with. Very few sociological ethnographers ever return to the same site for further explorations.

Nor is this the only way our consent procedures are flawed. Our disclosures about confidentiality and anonymity are likewise inadequate. Here, too, the problem lies more with what we do not say than with what we do. We routinely promise confidentiality and anonymity. Even when subjects have requested to be clearly identified or have had no objections to being identified, I have resisted. In part, I resist because confidentiality serves separate ends of my own. However much they protect subjects, confidentiality and anonymity are important rhetorical devices for ethnographic reportage. They transform the specific into the general. This surgical ward becomes the world of surgery. This blighted urban neighborhood becomes every urban neighborhood. Without confidentiality and anonymity, arguments about this transformation and about the representativeness that it effortlessly provides would be even more tedious and never-ending than they already are.

There is an irony, though, in our sincere promise of confidentiality and anonymity and in our clumsy efforts to achieve it. We succeed where it matters least and fail where it matters most. For those far from the scene, our pseudonyms effectively disguise the location of our investigations and the identity of our subjects. But then for these readers little would matter if we named actual names, because our subjects rarely are known outside local circles. But none of this is true in the actual community where the research was done. Here no attempt to disguise is ever wholly adequate. One could argue that this is a reason for multiple-site case studies. However, this solution compounds the problem rather than solves it. Subjects, and the colleagues of subjects, can read the ethnographer's writings, and this reading poses a real, if largely unacknowledged, risk to the research from the subject's point of view.

The risk is the one that Bill Smith recognized immediately, even if too late, when he first skimmed the text of *All God's Mistakes:* I said those things about my colleagues, but I didn't realize that they would see them. Now that they will, how can I continue to work with them? Not only was Smith's complaint justified, but I also should have anticipated it on the basis of my past experience. In *Forgive and Remember,* all of my attempts to conceal the identity of individuals and the organization failed most spectacularly at Pacific Hospital. To this day, the place where *Forgive and Remember* moves most briskly off the shelves is the Pacific University bookstore. The hospital staff there at all levels and from all departments read the book as a *roman à clef.* And this remains so despite the fact that with the passage of time, few of my original subjects are still at Pacific. Yet the readers on the Pacific payroll have no trouble figuring out who is who. For years, informants have told me that these successful decodings always provide a secret, guilty pleasure to readers: "Ah ha, so he really thought that." "That's just like him to behave that poorly." "Boy, I'm glad, I don't have to deal directly with that son of a bitch." Having failed so spectacularly at providing confidentiality and anonymity once before at the place were it was most necessary, I should have anticipated Bill Smith's objection.

The issue is deeper than a single unkept promise. The decoding of the text by locals has consequences; as Schutz (1962) was so fond of saying, it "gears into the world." Consider the data of most interest to members of the local institution: the airing of dirty laundry in public and statements about colleagues' behaviors made behind their back in the heat of a private moment. Such statements are like letters written in anger; but unlike such letters, they have been sent, received, and digested. Such statements also are similar to angry remarks directed to another in public. But unlike public remarks, they do not provide the opportunity to respond to a colleague's hurt feelings. Social life provides wiggle room; texts on social life do not. The very fact that such criticisms are made behind closed doors is an indicator that those making them did not want them displayed before an audience. When I am an audience of one for such "emotional flooding out," I use every means I know to keep the affect flowing. This means that the revelations that I make public often go further than subjects intended. Certainly, the text always contains more than subjects would reveal if I routinely said at such moments, "Are you sure you want to go there? Remember, I'm taking notes. Someday this all might appear in a book that your colleagues will be able to read."

There is, then, a very real risk that derives from the utter impossibility of maintaining confidentiality and anonymity at a local level. The atmosphere of naive trust that makes work possible is placed in jeopardy. The world becomes a less happy place. It is hard to know how to warn of these risks, because they share so little with the ordinary risks of social life. We frank postmoderns at the beginning of the twenty-first century place a high value on candor. Our subjects likely are to believe mistakenly that they are the kind of people who would never say anything in private that they would not say in public. They may even pride themselves on this self-deception to their later chagrin. All of this serves to illustrate that, as Goffman (1961) so epigrammatically and enigmatically put it in another context, "Life may not be much of a gamble, but interaction is." And Goffman forgot to add, "Interaction is a gamble against much longer odds when there is an ethnographer present."

Conclusion: Ethnographer-Ethicist Beware

Philosophers who advocate a more narrative, more deeply contextualized, more socially situated bioethics often point to the ethnographies of medical sociologists as examples of the kind of work they have in mind (Hoffmaster 1992). The implication is that if only ethicists either used or did more of this sort of work, if they only provided a "thicker description," then much of the ambiguity and uncertainty embedded in principlist approaches to bioethics would disappear.

This essay has been an oblique plea for philosophers to look elsewhere for help. The rationales offered have been largely pragmatic or emotional/moral. Ethnography invariably involves deception. Subjects misread the ethnographer's interest in their world, and ethnographers take no pains to correct these misreadings. Subjects do not understand that ethnographers debunk what Becker (1968) called "conventional sentimentality," the commonly accepted social versions of virtue and vice; that ethnographers write in an arch, ironic voice; that the objective of ethnographic writing often is to "debunk"; and that this debunking is accomplished by showing how altruistic statements hide self-interested motives. When subjects read what is written about them, they often feel betrayal. Beyond that, the doing of ethnography often rests on promises of confidentiality and anonymity that are invariably broken and, if not broken, at the very least are made without any confidence in or control over whether they will be kept.

These deceptions and broken promises ethnographers are willing to accept. As researchers, ethnographers are willing to apply a utilitarian calculus. The knowledge gained is worth the harm inflicted (at least as far as the researcher is concerned). And, if truth be told, these deceptions and broken promises are not usually a problem. The typical sociological ethnography focuses on those low in status hierarchies, those who command little respect, and those who are demonized by respectable society. Debunking in these circumstances means showing that those who might otherwise be thought of as moral monsters are really rational and honorable creatures, living within the rules of their subcultures. So, for such subjects, ethnography actually elevates their moral status. Because few of these subjects read our accounts, the potential for harm is minimal. However, all this changes when ethnographers study high-status groups. Debunking in this situation involves the ethnographer showing that those with noble social position are more base than commonly realized. Here, subjects are highly literate, and ethnographers can do harm in local settings where their work, if read, can destroy mutual trust. Unfortunately, this is a problem that is easier to identify than to remedy. Even so, as far as ethnographers are concerned, there is no other way to go about the research. If what the ethnographer writes is truthful—leaving to one side, for the moment, the complexities involved in making such an assessment—this is a defense all its own. If the shoe pinches, if the facts are inconvenient, that is what Weber (Gerth and Mills 1956) so long ago told us that science as a vocation was about.

But even if they satisfy social scientists, for ethicists these justifications are not wholly adequate. If one wishes to "do" ethics, there is an expectation that one will be above reproach. The manipulations, deceptions, evasions, and silences, without which it is impossible to gather data, make it hard for any ethnographer—no matter how pure his or her motivation, no matter how scrupulous his or her conduct—to be above reproach. In short, to produce a more narrative ethics, to introduce ethnographic methods into bioethics, may force the ethicist to act in ways that give lie to the claim, "I am an ethicist."

If ethicist were a role like ethnographer, that is to say, if the ethicist did research in one place and taught in another, then perhaps the moral failings embedded in the research process would not be of much moment. Alternatively, if ethicist were one of those roles where there was no expectation of a relationship between knowing and doing, then the betrayals and deceptions of the researcher would not count for much. But matters are not so simple. For ethicists, there is a role-based incompatibility between the doing of ethics and the doing of ethnography.

Since Simmel (Levine 1970), ethnographers often have claimed their unique purchase on social life is made possible because they are "strangers" to the scenes they explore. As such, they possess a paradoxical combination of nearness and distance, remoteness and intimacy. The world at hand, to lapse for a moment into phenomenological jargon, is both accessible and puzzling. Of course, by the end of an intensive fieldwork experience, the ethnographer is no longer a stranger. The world at hand is now familiar; its original mysteries are now nothing more than a set of everyday routines, contingent accomplishments, and repeated occurrences. More than anything else, it is this loss of stranger status for the fieldworker and of phenomenological puzzlement for the social world that explains the fact that sociological fieldworkers so often flit from site to site or topic to topic rather than continually try to mine the same settings. Gathering data as an ethnographer requires a certain skill at playing dumb; any reputation, however minimal, at being an expert or insider undermines the charade of social stupidity and thereby makes the research task that much more difficult. Beyond that, in solving the mysteries of any particular social world, the researcher develops relationships, makes friends, and builds obligations. This is so even though the fieldworker is a transient in the studied social world with no role to play once the research project is completed. The feelings that publication evokes among subjects then make it difficult to sustain those relationships, retain those friendships, and honor those obligations.

Unlike ethnographers, bioethicists are usually insiders in hospitals. As hospital employees, they sit on ethics committees, consult on difficult cases, teach medical students and residents, and provide a visible presence for ethics. In all this work, they, too, develop relationships, make friends, build obligations, and have a political stake in the organization. Hospital-based ethicists work in an environment in which strong norms of confidentiality exist. If bioethicists were to do ethnography, or even provide examples from their clinical experience of a more narrative version of ethics, they would need to trade on those relationships, betray some of those friendships, ignore some of those obligations, and tread, however lightly, on those norms of confidentiality. For bioethicists, the work of "displaying the data" might very well involve airing some dirty organizational linen that could transform insiders in hospitals to outsiders. This, then, may compromise the bioethicist's effectiveness as a front-line worker, as a committee member, as a consultant, as a teacher, and as a visible symbol of ethics.

Put most simply, if bioethicists themselves heed the call to produce a more contextual, a more narrative ethics, they may undercut their effectiveness in their other organizational roles. Studying some things one way makes it impossible to do other things in other ways. To that problem, we may add another. Full participation, a stake in outcomes, makes it difficult to achieve the distance that is part of what makes ethnographic interpretation possible. Partisan accounts often are detailed and very convincing, serve a purpose, and provide a unique window into a social world. They are many things; but one thing they are not is ethnography.

There is, of course, a difference between doing and using, creating and appreciating, making and applying. A more contextual bioethics does not require that bioethicists become ethnographers. But ethnography, as currently practiced by ethnographers, is not likely to produce accounts all that useful to bioethicists. For that to be so, ethnographers would need to be trained to take the normative as seriously as they take the empirical, to see the normative as something more substantial than a reflection of material interests and the cultural values associated with them. There is very little in social science theory or training that allows for this now. Nor are current trends any reason to feel sanguine about the future. Further, if ethnographers were to make the ethical dilemmas of the bedside the subject of their inquiries, then the everyday work of bioethicists would become the observational basis of their interpretive activities. This places bioethics in context to be sure; but it does so without necessarily producing an account of how the work of ethics is done that would be useful to bioethicists. After all, such accounts would be marked by that ironic and debunking tone that invariably creates tensions between ethnographers and their subjects.

REFERENCES

Anspach, Renee R. 1993. *Deciding Who Lives: Fateful Choices in the Intensive-Care Nursery.* Berkeley: University of California Press.

Becker, Howard. 1968. Whose Side Are We On? *Social Problems* 14:239–247.

Bluebond-Langer, Myra. 1978. *The Private Worlds of Dying Children.* Princeton, NJ: Princeton University Press.

Bosk, Charles L. 1979. *Forgive and Remember: Managing Medical Failure.* Chicago: University of Chicago Press.

———. 1992. *All God's Mistakes: Genetic Counseling in a Pediatric Hospital.* Chicago: University of Chicago Press.

Edin, Kathryn, and Laura Lein. 1997. *Making Ends Meet: How Single Mothers Survive Welfare and Low-Wage Work.* New York: Russell Sage Foundation.

Geertz, Clifford. 1973. *The Interpretation of Cultures.* New York: Basic Books.

Gerth, Hans, and C. W. Mills. 1956. *From Max Weber.* Glencoe, IL, and New York: Free Press.

Goffman, Erving. 1961. *Interaction Ritual.* New York: Pantheon.

Hoffmaster, Barry. 1992. Can Ethnography Save the Life of Medical Ethics? *Social Science and Medicine* 35:1421–1431.

Klockars, Carl. 1974. *The Professional Fence.* New York: Free Press.

Levine, Donald. 1971. *Georg Simmel: On Individuality and Social Forms.* Chicago: University of Chicago Press.

Park, Robert, and Ernest Burgess. [1922] 1967. *The City.* Chicago: University of Chicago Press.

Sanchez-Jankowski, Martin. 1991. *Islands in the Street: Gangs and American Urban Society.* Berkeley: University of California Press.

Schutz, Alfred. 1962. *The Collected Papers,* Vol. 1. The Hague: Martinus Nijhoff.

Van Maanen, John. 1988. *Tales of the Field: On Writing Ethnography.* Chicago: University of Chicago Press.

Whyte, William Foote. 1955. *Street Corner Society.* Chicago: University of Chicago Press.

Zussman, Robert. 1992. *Intensive Care: Medical Ethics and the Medical Profession.* Chicago: University of Chicago Press.

BARRY HOFFMASTER

Afterword

MANY OF the chapters in this volume employ qualitative research methods. Indeed, the use of such methods, ethnography in particular, seems to be central to creating the kind of contextual approach to bioethics that this volume seeks (see Conrad 1994; Hoffmaster 1992; Jennings 1990). That view has become almost commonplace, for as Fox and DeVries have observed, "Among sociologists working in the field of bioethics, it is taken for granted that the method par excellence of conducting socially and culturally cognizant and sensitive bioethical research is ethnography" (1998:273).

Bosk's list of ethnography's moral violations should, however, chasten those who advocate the contextualized, socially situated kind of bioethics that ethnography could help produce. But what exactly is the upshot of his argument? At times Bosk suggests that ethnography is so riven with moral problems that it ought to be abandoned. That is not Bosk's tempered view, though, for he believes that ethnography can be justified on pragmatic, utilitarian grounds. But if so, who should undertake it? Social scientists who are pragmatic and utilitarian would not have the requisite training or expertise in ethics. And bioethicists could not risk breaching confidentiality or proceeding without informed consent because those are precisely the kinds of moral failings to which bioethicists are attuned and which they are supposed to prevent. So to whom does one turn?

Bosk makes a compelling case that ethnography is morally dicey. That should be acknowledged, and ethnographers should be prepared for the moral perplexities and temptations they will encounter. Nevertheless, his case does not, in my view, entail that ethnography ought not to be done, or even that bioethicists morally (as opposed to prudentially) ought not to do it.

The ethnographic research reviewed in the introduction and contained in this volume is an important contribution to bioethics, and the value of this work does not depend upon any link to formal doctrines of bioethics or moral philosophy. Moreover, I doubt that the fieldworkers who conducted this research sought or actually obtained explicit training in ethics before embarking on their projects. And the contention that bioethicists cannot be utilitarians needs to be explained and defended. That claim cannot be conceptually true because Peter Singer, a renowned, albeit controversial, utilitarian, recently became the Ira W. DeCamp Professor of Bioethics at Princeton University (Specter 1999). Anyway, why could bioethicists who are not utilitarians be responsibly pragmatic, pragmatic in a way that permits them to do ethnography and still live with themselves even if they are not saints? But even if bioethicists were deterred by Bosk's warnings, informed, wary social scientists could continue to do ethnographic research. Bosk's more modest claim—that ethnography has moral and scientific limits—should, of course, be heeded, and consequently too much should not be expected of it. Within those limits, though, ethnography has the capacity to illuminate and advance bioethics, as it has done in many ways already.

What might be the philosophical implications of such qualitative work? Reviewing changes that have occurred over the first three decades of contemporary bioethics, Pellegrino observes, "Medical ethics is now increasingly a branch of moral philosophy" (1993:1158). Traditional moral philosophy is concerned with the justification of principles and decisions, and that justification ultimately derives from a rationally vindicated moral theory. The search for such a theory might be conducted in redoubtable foundationalist terms; that is, it might look for undeniable, unassailable fundamental axioms from which moral rules and judgments can be derived.[1] Or it might be conducted in more lenient, and currently more popular, coherentist terms. It might aim at a state of "reflective equilibrium," that is, maximal coherence of a set of considered moral judgments, moral principles, and background theories.[2] In either event, justification remains a matter of theory construction and deployment—an exercise in rational systematization.

How could the social sciences be related to the philosophical project of justification? Social science forays into bioethics might, on the one hand, produce information that can be used to improve and extend the ways in which moral theories and the principles they encompass or generate are brought to bear. This possibility is an instance of the "'good facts make good ethics' school of thought," that is, the stance that "the best descriptive work of ethnographers can provide a secure foundation for the best analytic, normative work of ethicists and moral philosophers" (Crigger 1995:400). Moral philosophy and the social sciences are, in this view, compatible and complementary. Yet the gulf between normative and descriptive, and the division of labor between philosophers and social scientists, remain intact.

On the other hand, the relationship might not be nearly that congenial. Qualitative research could, in various ways, raise doubts about the model of justification on which the analytic, normative work of ethicists and moral philosophers is predicated. The philosophical model of justification does not fit neatly or easily the phenomenology of moral deliberation and decision making that qualitative research reveals. It is hard to reconcile with Kaufman's exposure of the flux, ambiguity, and uncertainty of clinical-moral decision making and the multiple contexts within which that decision making is embedded; with Lock's analysis of the multiple bases for Japanese resistance to brain death; with Halpern's historical survey of shifting attitudes toward human experimentation; and with Conrad's accounts of how media depictions of bioethics problems can influence social understandings of and responses to those problems. Moral experience does not have the clarity, precision, and rigor, or the constancy and consistency that a moral theory requires, and those demands cannot be imposed on moral experience without substantial loss and distortion.

Nor does the philosophical model of justification neatly or easily accommodate the various roles that Anspach and Beeson attribute to the emotions in moral deliberation. Yet there are a variety of ways in which, as Elgin puts it, "emotions advance understanding" (1996:147).[3] Emotions heighten our awareness and direct our attention to matters that are morally salient. Emotions prompt us to recognize categories we have ignored and to reassess and reclassify behavior and attitudes. Emotions incite us to investigate and motivate us to persevere in those investigations. "Emotional honesty," as Elgin points out, "pays epistemic dividends": "In knowing how she feels about something, a subject knows what she thinks of it" (1996:160). To be sure, emotions can also impede moral understanding and undermine moral judgment. Emotions can generate wishful thinking that leads us astray, and the reactions induced by powerful emotions such as anger, terror, and infatuation can obliterate understanding. Emotions need to be scrutinized to sort out their positive and negative contributions to morality, but that is not a task amenable to justification by theory.

Moreover, there are independent worries about the standard philosophical approach to justification. Principally, justification by theory cannot succeed on its own terms because many moral issues arise and are settled beyond the confines of a moral theory.[4] Decisions have to be made, for example, about the domain of morality, that is, what entities fall within the ambit of morality and what status those entities have, and those decisions logically precede the application of moral norms or theories. For example, do anencephalic infants, babies born with a brain stem but little or no upper brain, have the full moral status of human beings, or are they special in a way that would permit transplantable organs to be retrieved from them even though they are not yet dead? As well, moral norms and theories are too abstract and general to be self-applying. Considerable moral work occurs in describing and characterizing situations so as to bring them within the purview of norms and theories. Is artificial nutrition and hydration, for instance, a form of medical treatment or basic, humane care? The moral classification of artificial nutrition and hydration will determine which norms are morally relevant and applicable rather than vice versa.

In addition, many of the substantive concepts of moral theory are thin and context dependent. A prime example of both is the notion of autonomy. Marshall's description of her ethics consultation with Faith shows that, although respect for Faith's autonomy protected her from undue pressure, it did not inform or guide her decision. In fact, respect for Faith's autonomy helped to put her in her excruciatingly difficult situation. Faith had to work her way through her agonizing plight largely on her own; understanding how she did that and how she could have been helped to do that should be where bioethics begins. And although the rationale for respecting autonomy is clear in acute care, it is not so clear in long-term or chronic care. It has been suggested, for example, that in long-term care

> we need to rethink the concept of autonomy, so central to bioethics in recent years. In the nursing home setting, because of the kinds of physical and mental limitations most residents face and because of the social functioning of a nursing home as an institution, autonomy and dependency cannot be seen as opposites. Instead, they must be seen as intertwined facets of one's life and one's state of being. Similarly, autonomy and community must be made mutually compatible in a nursing home setting if we are to get a full and realistic moral purchase on how life is actually lived there. (Collopy, Boyle, and Jennings 1991:3)

Moral concepts and norms must fit the settings and the circumstances in which they are invoked, but determining whether they are contextually appropriate again takes one beyond the terms of standard moral theory.

There is a practical worry here, too. As Caplan (1983) emphasized some time ago, effectiveness in bioethics is more likely to be a matter of creative problem solving than theoretical justification. One of Caplan's notable successes was resolving a problem of scarce resources in a hospital emergency room. Every summer people suffering from emphysema and other respiratory ailments would crowd the emergency room in hot weather for the oxygen they needed to breathe comfortably. Because there were only two oxygen units available, the staff of the emergency room asked Caplan to help them devise fair, equitable criteria for allocating their scarce medical resource. Caplan dutifully read the philosophical and theological literature about ethics and microallocation. Then he had an inspiration. He asked whether Medicaid/Medicare would provide air conditioners in the homes of patients with respiratory ailments. To everyone's surprise, they could be prescribed and the cost reimbursed. Caplan became an instant "moral guru" (1983:312). The lesson he draws is that "ethical theory would have been the wrong place to turn for a solution" (1983:312). Understanding and investigating the circumstances in which the problem arose turned out to be the right place.

Finally, the requirement of justification by theory makes bioethics a rather exclusive professional club. It remains an enclave for those who have special academic training and special theoretical expertise. Those who live through the problems these specialists analyze and debate—the people whom Beeson and Doksum interviewed and the nurses whom McBurney watched try to engage their ethics committee—continue to be ignored and silent.

Too much of morality escapes the rational systematization that yields a moral theory. The focus of that enterprise is too narrow, and its terms are too constraining. Moving beyond the philosophical approach to moral justification does not mean, however, that rationality has no role to play in morality or bioethics. But it is a different conception of rationality, one better exemplified by judgment than by justified decision. It is captured by Nussbaum's description of a kind of Aristotelian moral deliberation: "[T]he only procedure to follow is . . . to imagine all the relevant features as well and fully and concretely as possible, holding them up against whatever intuitions and emotions and plans and imaginings we have brought into the situation or can construct in it" (1990:74).[5] As Nussbaum emphasizes, this kind of deliberation makes room for the personal and the creative: "Good deliberation is like theatrical or musical improvisation, where what counts is flexibility, responsiveness, and openness to the external. . . . It is possible to play a jazz solo from a score, making minor alterations for the particular nature of one's instrument. The question is, who would do this, and why?" (1990:74).

Rather than being a largely abstract endeavor, moral philosophy needs to attend more closely and more carefully to the times, the places, the structures, and the circumstances within which moral problems arise and to the people for whom they are problems. Moral philosophy also has to reconcile the objective demands of reason that make matters of morality matters of principle with the subjective personal judgment that is the source of both moral freedom and moral responsibility. In pursuing those goals, moral philosophy needs to draw upon and incorporate the insights of the social sciences. That is the way toward a conception of morality that does not segregate reason and experience, philosophers and social scientists, but rather assimilates them in ways that are more practically helpful and more philosophically tenable.

NOTES

1. This, for example, is the approach of Peter Singer, who ends up with a utilitarian moral theory. See Singer 1974 and 1993.

2. This becomes the approach of Beauchamp and Childress in the fourth edition of *Principles of Biomedical Ethics* (1994). The notion of reflective equilibrium comes from Rawls 1971, but its development is elaborated in Daniels 1996.

3. The points in this paragraph are taken from Elgin 1996, ch. V.

4. This point is made in Hoffmaster 1994. The underlying problem is the notion of formal reason embedded in the philosophical project of theory construction. That problem is more clearly articulated in an unpublished version of this paper presented at the International Working Conference on Non-Formal Foundations of Reason, held in Newcastle, New South Wales, Australia, August 1–6, 1993.

5. A strength of this account is that it accords with how people actually seem to make decisions, at least in some contexts. For example, women struggling to make decisions after reproductive counseling reject the official "maximize subjective expected utility" approach in favor of an approach along the lines Nussbaum describes. See Hoffmaster 1991.

References

Beauchamp, Tom L., and James F. Childress. 1994. *Principles of Biomedical Ethics,* 4th ed. New York: Oxford University Press.

Caplan, Arthur L. 1983. Can Applied Ethics Be Effective in Health Care and Should It Strive to Be? *Ethics* 93:311–319.

Collopy, Bart, Philip Boyle, and Bruce Jennings. 1991. New Directions in Nursing Home Ethics. *Hastings Center Report* (Suppl.) 21(2):1–16.

Conrad, Peter. 1994. How Ethnography Can Help Bioethics. *Bulletin of Medical Ethics* May:13–18.

Crigger, Bette-Jane. 1995. Bioethnography: Fieldwork in the Lands of Medical Ethics. *Medical Anthropology Quarterly* 9:400–417.

Daniels, Norman. 1996. *Justice and Justification.* Cambridge: Cambridge University Press.

Elgin, Catherine Z. 1996. *Considered Judgment.* Princeton, NJ: Princeton University Press.

Fox, Renee C., and Raymond DeVries. 1998. Afterword: The Sociology of Bioethics. In *Bioethics and Society,* eds. Raymond DeVries and Janardan Subedi, 270–276. Upper Saddle River, NJ: Prentice Hall.

Hoffmaster, Barry. 1991. The Theory and Practice of Applied Ethics. *Dialogue* 30:213–234.

———. 1992. Can Ethnography Save the Life of Medical Ethics? *Social Science and Medicine* 35:1421–1431.

———. 1994. The Forms and Limits of Medical Ethics. *Social Science and Medicine* 39:1155-1164.

Jennings, Bruce. 1990. Ethics and Ethnography in Neonatal Intensive Care. In *Social Science Perspectives on Medical Ethics,* ed. George Weisz, 261–272. Boston: Kluwer Academic.

Nussbaum, Martha C. 1990. *Love's Knowledge.* New York: Oxford University Press.

Pellegrino, Edmund D. 1993. The Metamorphosis of Medical Ethics. *JAMA* 269:1158–1162.

Rawls, John. 1971. *A Theory of Justice.* Cambridge, MA: Harvard University Press.

Singer, Peter. 1974. Sidgwick and Reflective Equilibrium. *The Monist* 58:490–517.

———. 1993. *Practical Ethics,* 2nd ed. Cambridge: Cambridge University Press.

Specter, Michael. 1999. The Dangerous Philosopher. *The New Yorker* 75 (Sept. 6):46–55.

About the Contributors

RENEE R. ANSPACH is Associate Professor of Sociology and Women's Studies at the University of Michigan. Her work on the sociology of bioethics and medical sociology includes the award-winning *Deciding Who Lives: Fateful Choices in the Intensive-Care Nursery.*

DIANE BEESON is Professor of Sociology and Chair of the Department of Sociology and Social Services at California State University, Hayward. Her articles have appeared in the *Journal of Medical Genetics, Journal of Genetic Counseling, Social Problems, Sociological Perspectives,* and various anthologies.

CHARLES L. BOSK is a professor in the Department of Sociology, a faculty associate at the Center of Bioethics, and a senior fellow of The Leonard Davis Institute at the University of Pennsylvania. He is the author of *Forgive and Remember: Managing Medical Failure* and *All God's Mistakes: Genetic Counseling in a Pediatric Hospital.*

PETER CONRAD is the Harry Coplan Professor of Social Sciences and Chair of the Department of Sociology at Brandeis University. He has written or edited a dozen books, including the award-winning *Deviance and Medicalization: From Badness to Sickness.*

TERESA DOKSUM is an associate at Abt Associates Inc. in Cambridge, Massachusetts. Her articles have appeared in *Genetics in Medicine, Community Genetics, Obstetrics and Gynecology,* and several oncology journals.

SYDNEY A. HALPERN is Associate Professor of Sociology at the University of Illinois at Chicago. She is the author of *American Pediatrics: The Social Dynamics of Professionalism, 1880–1980* and *Moral Communities in Medical Science: Early Vaccine Use and the Problem of Risk* (2001).

BARRY HOFFMASTER is a professor in the Department of Philosophy and the Department of Family Medicine at the University of Western Ontario. He is a coauthor of *Ethical Issues in Family Medicine* and a coeditor of *Health Care Ethics in Canada.*

SHARON R. KAUFMAN is Professor in Residence in the Department of Social and Behavioral Science and the Department of Anthropology, History and Social Medicine at the University of California, San Francisco. She is the author of *The Ageless Self: Sources of Meaning in Late Life* and *The Healer's Tale: Transforming Medicine and Culture.*

MARGARET LOCK is a professor in the Department of Social Studies of Medicine and the Department of Anthropology at McGill University. She is the author of the prize-winning *Encounters with Aging: Mythologies of Menopause in Japan and North America* and *Twice Dead: Organ Transplants and the Reinvention of Death.*

PATRICIA A. MARSHALL is the Associate Director of Medical Humanities and an associate professor of medicine in the Stritch School of Medicine at Loyola University of Chicago. She is a coeditor of *Clinical Medical Ethics: Cases and Readings* and *Integrating Cultural, Observational, and Epidemiological Approaches in the Prevention of Drug Abuse and HIV/AIDS.*

CATE MCBURNEY has several years' experience as a clinical ethicist and is currently a doctoral candidate in bioethics at the University of Montreal. Her research interests include the contributions of the social sciences to bioethics and ethical issues at the end of life, especially related to pain control and the use of advance directives.

Index